Psychology in Diabetes Care and Practice

This is an indispensable guide to diabetes care and practice, providing a thorough overview of the main issues that health professionals should keep in mind when treating someone with the condition, and how psychology plays a key role in diabetes self-management.

Based on the latest research evidence along with numerous patient perspectives, the book looks at a wide range of topics in diabetes health psychology, from mental health conditions to theories of behaviour change, with a focus on comorbidities. Chapters describe the emotional impact of a diabetes diagnosis; the psychosocial issues surrounding living with diabetes; theories of behaviour applied to diabetes self-management; the impact of diabetes and depression; diabetes and eating disorders; the psychological impact of diabetes complications, and potential stigma associated with having Type 2 diabetes, including the psychological impact of weight loss surgery.

Psychology in Diabetes Care and Practice enables the provision of support to reduce psychological distress and improve diabetes self-management. It helps patients to learn more about how best to manage their condition, as well as health professionals wanting to find appropriate ways to facilitate self-management.

Dr Val Wilson is an academic with a PhD in diabetes health education from the University of Kent, UK. As a specialist in the field, she has conducted various research studies about how people self-manage their diabetes over the past 25 years. She has also carried out more than ten years of voluntary work with the INPUT (Insulin Pump Therapy) national diabetes organisation. Dr Wilson has published widely in nursing and healthcare journals and has had Type 1 diabetes for 45 years.

Psychology in Diabetes Care and Practice

Dr. Val Wilson

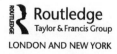 Routledge
Taylor & Francis Group

LONDON AND NEW YORK

First published 2022
by Routledge
2 Park Square, Milton Park, Abingdon, Oxon OX14 4RN

and by Routledge
605 Third Avenue, New York, NY 10158

Routledge is an imprint of the Taylor & Francis Group, an informa business

© 2022 Val Wilson

British Library Cataloguing-in-Publication Data
A catalogue record for this book is available from the British Library

Library of Congress Cataloguing-in-Publication Data
Names: Wilson, Val, 1967- author.
Title: Psychology in diabetes care and practice / Val Wilson.
Description: Milton Park, Abingdon, Oxon ; New York, NY :
Routledge, 2022.
Identifiers: LCCN 2021040958 (print) | LCCN 2021040959
(ebook) | ISBN 9781032196473 (paperback) | ISBN
9781032196497 (hardback) | ISBN 9781003260219 (ebook)
Subjects: LCSH: Diabetes--Psychological aspects.
Classification: LCC RC660 .W55 2022 (print) | LCC RC660
(ebook) | DDC 616.4/620651--dc23/eng/20211013
LC record available at https://lccn.loc.gov/2021040958
LC ebook record available at https://lccn.loc.gov/2021040959

ISBN: 978-1-032-19649-7 (hbk)
ISBN: 978-1-032-19647-3 (pbk)
ISBN: 978-1-003-26021-9 (ebk)

DOI: 10.4324/9781003260219

Typeset in Bembo
by MPS Limited, Dehradun

For Neil

Contents

Introduction

Diabetes mellitus occurs when there is a change in the way the body is able to use glucose as fuel, causing there to be an increase in blood glucose due to a lack of insulin to correct this imbalance. The condition has two main types: Type 1 diabetes, where insulin is no longer produced; and Type 2 diabetes, where there is increased insulin production to correct high blood glucose levels, but this cannot be used effectively by the body. Diabetes now presents health services with a huge challenge in terms of provision and cost as prevalence of the condition has escalated in recent years. The rise in cases of Type 2 diabetes – which accounts for 90 percent of all diagnoses – occurs in the majority of individuals due to a diet high in refined carbohydrates in combination with a sedentary lifestyle, signifying the worldwide increase in diabetes this century.

The psychological effects of diabetes have been identified and characterised for over thirty years. Research shows that the impact of diabetes on mental health increases in accordance with duration of the condition as the burden of diabetes and its complications increases (Hoban, et al, 2015; Ducat, et al, 2014). Burns (2001) suggests that when an individual has a physical condition or accident affecting health, this also damages self-concept, forcing a mentality of, 'Why me?'. Individuals must assess the degree to which their health condition impacts on their life and new approaches, activities, attitudes and social relationships are constructed. This is addressed by attempting to reduce the impact of a health condition with behaviour change interventions, although Burns states that it is not sufficient to advise that an individual learns to cope with a physical or psychological condition by adjusting to their circumstances and accepting change.

A number of serious secondary complications can occur as a result of having continually abnormal glucose levels, such as heart and circulatory system disorders, and nerve, eye and kidney disease. Diabetes is a

DOI: 10.4324/9781003260219-1

complex metabolic disorder requiring the individual to continually self-manage blood glucose and cholesterol levels. This means that the individual must learn to monitor their condition so blood glucose levels are kept as close to a non-diabetic range as possible to minimise the risk of these further health problems. Diabetes is therefore unlike any other chronic health condition, as it is necessary for the individual to deliver more than 95 percent of their own care.

Demands such as consistent monitoring of blood glucose, administering insulin, taking oral medications, regular physical activity, and healthy eating may be overwhelming, with an additional psychological and social impact if diabetes complications are present. *The Future of Diabetes Report* showed that 64 percent of people with diabetes said that the condition affects them psychologically, while fewer than a quarter of people receive the emotional and psychological support they need from the NHS. For this reason, healthcare professionals must recognise how and why psychosocial factors shape the way individuals care for their condition. From diagnosis, personal health beliefs, health goals and motivations influence diabetes self-care and self-management behaviour; this is subject to change as duration of the condition increases.

The impact of psychosocial issues on individuals with diabetes became more prominent with the publication of the *National Service Framework (NSF) for Diabetes: Standards* document (Department of Health, 2003a). NSF Standard 3 highlights the need for those with diabetes to receive structured health education and psychological support to assist self-management of the condition; this standard envisioned that appropriate health education and support would enable individuals to engage in diabetes self-care to the best extent achievable. The need for patient-centred psychological care for those with diabetes has been widely documented (Titchner, 2020; Sanne, et al., 2019; Ham, et al.; 2017; Williams, et al., 2016). However, *The Future of Diabetes Report* showed that little had changed since Wilson (2003a) conducted a survey revealing that 92 percent of 155 people with diabetes did not have a psychologist or trained counsellor as part of their diabetes team. In the 15-year gap between surveys, the need for psychological support for people with diabetes remained – and continues to be – unmet due to poor availability via the NHS.

Although it has been reported that £25,000 is spent on diabetes every minute in the UK, with £14 billion per annum spent on complications (diabetes.co.uk, 2019), four-fifths of this expenditure goes on medication and surgical procedures rather than providing counselling. Recently, COVID-19 is taking an emotional toll across the world, with rising levels of mental ill-health after living with uncertainty and disruption for many months, putting a great strain on mental health services generally. The issue of sparse psychological support for people with diabetes is therefore set to continue as NHS funding in the United Kingdom is stretched to capacity.

Obesity carries with it the risk of developing Type 2 diabetes, which is 80 times greater than for the non-obese (Abdullah, et al., 2011); the number of adults and children becoming obese and going on to develop Type 2 diabetes is steadily rising due to lifestyle factors (Yanling, et al., 2016; Temneanu, et al., 2016). A diagnosis of diabetes brings with it not only physical consequences, but also a huge psychological impact affecting the individual and everyone around them. This burden includes:

- Coping with the initial diagnosis.
- Awareness of and measures to prevent potential secondary complications if blood glucose levels are not well-controlled – such as blindness, kidney failure, amputation, stroke, and heart disease.
- Cognitive effects – the process of gaining knowledge about diabetes, including perceptions and reasoning.
- The psychological factors influenced by the condition, such as depression.

'I was frightened to death when blindness was mentioned because my grandmother had Type 2 diabetes, and she lost her sight'.

'When I developed Type 1 as an adult, I bought a couple of books about the condition. Images of amputated limbs and huge leg ulcers were difficult to process – I thought that it couldn't happen to me'.

'My whole life seems to have been taken over by diabetes and I hate it'.

The Department of Health *National Service Framework for Diabetes* (Department of Health, 2003) states that diabetes self-management is the key to good diabetes care. The document suggests that this can be achieved by the individual with the provision of information, education and psychological support from diabetes healthcare professionals:

"People with diabetes need the knowledge, skills and motivation to assess their risks, to understand what they will gain from changing their behaviour or lifestyle, and to act on that understanding by engaging in appropriate behaviours."

Although these guidelines exist and there is recognition by healthcare professionals and Government that people with diabetes require psychological support, it is important to determine why these needs are often overlooked in clinical practice (Li, et al., 2010; Pouwer, et al., 2006).

The *Diabetes and Emotional Health* handbook (Diabetes UK, 2019) suggests that little progress has been made due to healthcare professionals citing a lack of time, skills, confidence and availability of practical resources in this area. Therefore, existing guidelines acknowledge that there is a need for psychological support, but – with the exception of the *Diabetes and Emotional Health* handbook – there is a distinct lack of guidance for implementation in daily practice.

About this book

Psychology in Diabetes Care and Practice is aimed at healthcare professionals, providing up-to-date evidence and an overview of the main issues to keep in mind when treating someone with diabetes. Dr Val Wilson is a specialist in diabetes health education, having been involved in diabetes research for almost three decades, including more than ten years of voluntary work with the INPUT (Insulin Pump Therapy) national diabetes organisation. Dr Wilson has conducted numerous independent studies concerning how people self-manage their diabetes in different settings, and this book contains anonymous quotes to illustrate the individual's perspective of the issues highlighted in each chapter. As someone with a 45-year duration of Type 1 diabetes that is difficult to manage (brittle), Dr Wilson brings the long-term experience and insight of someone living with diabetes to *Psychology in Diabetes Care and Practice*.

In the opening two chapters, this book covers the emotional impact of a diabetes diagnosis, and the multitude of psychosocial issues affecting people with diabetes on a day-to-day basis; it is not as simple as just following the advice of healthcare professionals in order to manage the condition effectively. Having depression, for example, means that diabetes is more difficult to self-manage as depression leads to increased blood glucose levels, often with a reduction in the individual's ability to carry out self-care activities. Chapter three explores the theories behind how diabetes care is delivered, including how this care must be tailored according to individual circumstances.

Depression and eating disorders are discussed in Chapter four. The brain is continually influenced by chemical processes and fluctuating blood glucose levels that have a significant impact on how diabetes is self-managed in terms of thoughts, decisions and subsequent health-related behaviours. Emotions also play an intrinsic central role in consciousness and awareness, influencing the thoughts and activities expressed in decision making and subsequent behaviour. The individual can alter these behavioural and emotional influences by using techniques that increase awareness of activities that are unconducive to health. This can lead to a number of health benefits over time as changes occur in the way the individual thinks and reacts to challenges such as pain and depression. It may not be possible to control and manage Type 1 diabetes well if the condition is brittle. Chapter five explores disordered eating behaviour, which presents a greater challenge if the individual is attempting to lose weight, maintain weight loss, or as a control mechanism in order to cope with life events. The perspective of individuals who have faced these issues is included.

Type 1 diabetes is a condition where the immune system continually attacks the insulin-producing cells of the pancreas, generating antibodies that destroy these cells. Coexisting autoimmune conditions are common, such as asthma, psoriasis, coeliac disease, and thyroid disorders. These auto-immunities are explored in Chapter six, along with diabetes comorbidities, such as hypertension and dyslipidaemia. The individual must then manage multiple chronic health conditions, often presenting increasing problems with diabetes control. These issues are explored in Chapter six, with supporting quotes from individuals who have experienced these challenges.

With behavioural changes, Type 2 diabetes – often related to a high-carbohydrate diet and sedentary lifestyle – can be greatly improved or even reversed. With its huge toll on healthcare resources, much research has focused on reversing Type 2 diabetes using surgical weight loss techniques, enabling insulin to function normally in the body once more. However, weight loss surgery is not a quick fix and is frequently accompanied by a number of psychological issues that must be addressed. Stigma of having Type 2 diabetes and the expectations and challenges of those attempting to reverse the condition is examined in the final chapter of *Psychology in Diabetes Care and Practice*.

1 Diagnosis, Diabetes, and Emotional Impact

Currently, the total number of individuals with diabetes worldwide stands at 415,000,000, which is 1 in every 11 adults; this figure is estimated to rise to 642 million people living with diabetes by 2040. It is also estimated that 46 percent of people presently have undiagnosed diabetes (diabetes.co.uk, 2019). In the UK alone, 3.5 million people have diabetes of one form or other, the majority being diagnosed with Type 2 diabetes due to a sedentary lifestyle and a diet rich in unrefined carbohydrates. For UK children and teens under 20 years of age, the National Institute for Health (2017) reported that 208,000 young people now have either Type 1 or Type 2 diabetes. These statistics show the rate at which diabetes is rapidly increasingly, with many more cases still undiagnosed. A diabetes diagnosis has far-reaching consequences, affecting every individual both physically and psychologically.

Impact of a diabetes diagnosis

'It was a complete shock to be told I had Type 1 diabetes and what that would mean for the rest of my life. I didn't take it all in for months'.

'I couldn't believe what my doctor was telling me – that this illness had to be managed for the rest of my life, with a high risk of blindness and kidney failure if I didn't'.

'I refused to believe it when I was told I now have Type 2 diabetes. I didn't even feel ill and it was only found because of a routine blood test'.

DOI: 10.4324/9781003260219-2

Being diagnosed with diabetes may bring with it many negative emotions, such as shock, disbelief, fear, anger, distress and self-blame, although understanding what has been causing certain symptoms can also bring a sense of surprise and relief. It may be the case that there have been no symptoms at all, and the condition is discovered by chance. Similar to the bereavement response, the individual will go through stages such as anger, immobilisation, denial, bargaining, and acceptance as they come to terms with having a chronic, life-changing health condition. This realisation has been termed, 'the beginning of a new reality' (Diabetes UK, 2019).

Clinically, Type 1 diabetes onset – where there is ongoing auto-immune destruction of the insulin-producing cells of the pancreas – presents with acute hyperglycaemia, excessive thirst and urination. Often, ketoacidosis is present – where excess glucose cannot be used as fuel by the body and the blood becomes acidic, with the presence of ketone bodies. A diagnosis of Type 1 can follow other periods of illness, such as pancreatitis and more recently, COVID-19 with the diagnosis almost always being 'considered devastating' (Diabetes UK, 2019), despite the current availability of treatment technologies to enable a healthy life with the condition.

Type 2 diabetes presents far more slowly than Type 1, sometimes taking up to 12 years before the individual – perhaps after a long period of denial – reports symptoms such as increased thirst and urination to gain a diagnosis (Diabetes UK, 2008). Despite this slow onset, Type 2 diabetes is a complex metabolic condition caused by a variable degree of insulin resistance and/or defects in pancreatic insulin secretion, where complications such as heart disease and background retinopathy have already begun. It is wrong to think that Type 2 diabetes is not as serious as Type 1, nor that it only occurs in older people. There is a growing incidence of Type 2 diabetes in children and young adults, due to a diet high in refined carbohydrates and little or no exercise; Type 2 is also more predominant in children with a family history of the condition, and racial minorities such as Southeast Asians, Native Americans, Pacific Islanders or African Americans (Wilson, 2019).

Following a diabetes diagnosis, it is important that the individual:

- Understands the seriousness of their condition and the outcome if it is not properly managed.
- Is aware that if diabetes is managed as well as possible, complications are not inevitable. N.B. It should be noted that brittle Type 1 diabetes is not easy to manage, no matter how hard the individual tries.

- Know that having diabetes is accompanied by changeable emotions, such as depression, which can be treated if recognised and reported.

It is well known that individuals with either Type 1 or Type 2 diabetes mellitus experience a reduced feeling of psychological wellbeing because of the condition (Diabetes UK, 2019; Wilson, 2019). Perhaps as many as 50 percent of individuals being diagnosed with diabetes already have a feeling of adverse psychological wellbeing (Chew, et al., 2014; Walker, et al., 2012). This is due to high blood glucose levels creating chemical changes in the brain resulting in poor coping ability for other life events, such as work or family concerns disrupting the individual's daily routine prior to a diabetes diagnosis (Stuckey, et al., 2014).

Having diabetes can have a negative impact on the individual and their life, not just regarding disease self-management. The Diabetes Attitudes, Wishes and Needs second survey – DAWN2 – assessed the level of depression in 1,600 individuals with diabetes as 13.8 percent; diabetes-related distress as 44.6 percent; and perceived quality of life as 12.2 percent (Nicolucci, et al., 2013). The researchers reported that 20.5 percent of the individuals in the DAWN2 study agreed diabetes adversely affected their relationship with family and friends; 60.2 percent mentioned that diabetes negatively affected their physical health; and 40.0 percent felt diabetes medication disrupted their life to the extent that it was a problem. As a result, many people relied on negative coping strategies – such as smoking or over-eating – with the perception that their diabetes would definitely cause them problems in the future. If psychological issues go untreated, there is a marked association with poor physical health as a consequence (Bener, et al., 2012); cardiovascular disease (Laake, et al., 2014); and depressive symptoms (Diabetes UK, 2019).

Depression – whether diabetes-related or not – may lead to cognitive decline and can adversely affect the individual's ability to carry out diabetes self-care activities, so many studies have focused on major depressive disorder in diabetes (Park, et al., 2013; Sullivan, et al., 2013). However, psychological symptoms such as anxiety, stress and distress are more prevalent than major depressive disorder (Diabetes UK, 2019). These psychological disorders are associated with increased disability; steadily declining health; an increased use of healthcare facilities such as hospital appointments for eye and foot clinics, and a greater risk of early death (Goldney, et al., 2004). Older people with diabetes often have comorbidities that impair cognitive functioning, such as dementia, hypertension and cardiovascular disease. Age, duration of illness, diabetes complications, and poor glycaemic control may further complicate the relationship between cognitive function and diabetes.

> 'At my last diabetes clinic appointment, I told them I'd been diagnosed with depression and that I was taking an anti-depressant [Amitriptyline] with the side effect of increased blood sugar levels. There was absolutely no understanding or practical advice about this whatsoever'.
>
> 'My diabetes consultant and nurse don't have the time to offer any support. I'm just weighed, have my blood pressure and blood glucose measured, then a quick five-minute chat with the consultant for him to ask if anything's changed. I then get told to come back in a year'.
>
> 'I've never received any information from my diabetes team, not even a leaflet'.

The NHS Plan (NHS, 2000) states that too many patients feel talked about, rather than listened to. This suggests that many people do not consider themselves to be part of their diabetes team, their needs remaining uncommunicated and unmet. While those with diabetes are now invited to participate in diabetes care decisions, this should also address emotional, social, behavioural and psychological, as well as medical challenges. The *National Service Framework* (NSF) priorities for diabetes care document (Department of Health, 2002) states that 'all individuals with diabetes should be provided with educational and psychological support with the aim of facilitating and supporting self-management'. It is clear from the previous recent examples that this is not necessarily the case in practice.

What Diabetes Care to Expect (Diabetes UK, 2000) suggests that the individual should work with their healthcare team as an equal to achieve the best diabetes management. This implies ability and opportunity to communicate in a two-way discussion about diabetes management so the individual can make decisions and ask for what they need; additionally, the individual spends less than two hours a year with their diabetes team – everything else is self-management.

The *What Diabetes Care to Expect* patient information pamphlet gives a list of diabetes care team members including a psychologist, ophthalmologist, chiropodist, and dietician. Although being able to request emotional and psychological support is one of the 15 health checks in diabetes care (Diabetes UK, 2018), it may not be the norm – in practice, there is a distinct lack of available psychological support for individuals with diabetes due to NHS budgeting. A 2003 survey of 200 individuals across the UK with Type 1 diabetes showed that only 12 – representing 8 percent of participants – agreed that they could be referred to a psychologist or counsellor if needed (Wilson, 2003). Furthermore, just over half of the participants were unaware they could ask for psychological support if they had mental health issues affecting diabetes self-management. Little has changed in recent times.

'A mental health specialist should be part of the [diabetes] team to provide emotional support. I recently asked for this, but was told no support was available. I've never received any mental health support from my diabetes team – I'm not sure it ever existed. I only see the consultant and the nurse and that's the extent of my care team'.

'I was told that if my depression affected my blood glucose levels, then I could see a psychologist through my diabetes team. I was assessed by the nurse as managing OK because I still tested my blood regularly for my own benefit with complications, so my depression was labelled as non-diabetes related. I was advised to pay to see a counsellor privately, i.e. not an NHS mental health specialist with diabetes expertise'.

Diabetes and altered brain function

Brain function is modified by a number of significant factors, such as education, mood, age, blood flow, and metabolic fluctuations (Cranston, 2005), meaning this function differs within the individual and across populations over time. Research shows that having diabetes alters the brain both structurally and functionally (Chew, et al., 2014). Neurochemical changes in the regions of the brain controlling cognition increase the risk of depression in people with either Type 1 or Type 2 diabetes (Lyoo, et al., 2012). Impairment of neurons has been seen in people with diabetes mellitus due to abnormal glucose metabolism, resulting in poor maintenance of memory and learning, and an inability to control the expression of emotions (Giacco and Brownlee, 2010).

While there are many negative associations between diabetes and poor self-care, not all emotional consequences are negative; many individuals report a developed ability for self-awareness, self-confidence, hope and humour. Identifying and reflecting on good experiences can have immediate and lasting benefits that encourage motivation for self-care.

Inflammatory changes throughout the body of newly-diagnosed adults with Type 2 diabetes have been correlated with depressive symptoms (Laake, et al., 2014). This demonstrates the effect of negative mood on the immune system. It has been recognised that hyperglycaemia is very damaging to the body as it leads to oxidative stress – when cells die or are damaged beyond repair (Fiorentino, et al., 2013). Three factors contribute to oxidative stress: abnormally high HbA1c levels; the unstable nature of blood glucose levels in diabetes; and glucose swings from normal to very high incurred after meals. This cell destruction is responsible for vascular complications (Monnier, et al., 2006), while long-term high blood glucose levels cause perpetual cell breakdown, reducing mitochondrial DNA function (Hammes, 2003).

Other proteins and fats in the body are also subject to this degeneration due to high blood glucose levels (Aronson, 2008). Damage to the brain and blood vessels occurs when the individual with diabetes has high blood pressure and high levels of damaging blood fats, such as cholesterol. The breakdown of proteins into glucose – glycosylation – and the oxidation of cholesterol increases atherosclerosis – fatty deposits inside the arteries (Taguchi, et al., 2007).

There is a clear relationship between glycosylated haemoglobin (HbA1c) variations and the risk of stroke and heart disease in those with Type 2 diabetes, while variability in fasting blood glucose levels is linked to macro- and microvascular complications (Hirakawa, et al., 2014). Marked variation in HbA1c can cause nephropathy to worsen more significantly than if HbA1c is usually average; elevated HbA1c is also associated with the development and progression of retinopathy (Penno, et al., 2013). It is the case that the development of diabetic eye and kidney disease often occurs simultaneously. Erratic swings in blood glucose are not specifically highlighted in an HbA1c test because the lows and highs form an average amount of glucose sticking to the red blood cells over three months. Erratic glucose levels are a predictor of stroke, cardiovascular complications and mortality (Nalysnyk, et al., 2010).

For individuals with hypertension managed with medication, variations in systolic blood pressure are associated with a significant risk of vascular events, such as blocked arteries and stroke (Rothwell, et al., 2010); ongoing fluctuations in systolic blood pressure are strongly associated with the likelihood of stroke and heart attacks. Systolic blood pressure variations in younger individuals are a strong predictor of circulatory system complications, but this is associated with blood glucose levels rather than high cholesterol levels in those with diabetes.

> 'My daughter had a severe hypoglycaemic coma when she was 10 years old. Her brain function was permanently impaired, leaving her with epilepsy and learning disabilities'.

The brain relies on a constant supply of glucose for fuel, therefore it is to be expected that brain function can be drastically altered during hypo- or hyperglycaemia; too much glucose in the blood is toxic to the brain. The extent of these changes has been a research focus for decades, although more investigation is necessary. Many cerebral mechanisms are now better understood (Klein and Waxman, 2003) and continuing research aims to identify the impact of molecular changes causing defective cognitive and cerebral function in diabetes.

How an emotional response is formed

Emotions play a key role in consciousness and awareness; neurobiological and neuropsychological actions influence thoughts and activities which are then expressed in decision making and behaviour. Far from being separate functions, emotion and cognition are both interactive and integrated parts of the brain; this is consistent with the high degree of connectivity with brain structures and systems. As the relationship between emotion and cognition is well established, it can be seen that emotion directly affects cognition and behaviour when the individual's situation is personally or socially important to them.

Fear is a practical emotion: basic emotions – such as anger or fear – are evolutionary responses; more complex emotions, such as cognitions, perceptions and beliefs are personal to individuals and cultures. A basic emotional response is a subconscious reaction to an acute situation, while more complex emotional responses are processed using perception, intuition and reasoning. Thus, emotions act as a store for learned experiences, unique to individuals, ages, groups and cultures.

Several human behaviours are formed by the association between cognition and emotion, such as regulation – the desire to appropriately self-manage diabetes. Behaviour is more complex than solely being driven by emotion, although basic emotion always heralds behavioural action, as well as thoughts and action in response to more complex emotions (Izard, 2009). The influence of emotions on producing and altering behaviour depends on the type of emotion and the situation by which it arose; more complex emotions can result in action via its impact on cognition. Therefore, thinking guides and regulates behaviour evolving from complex emotions. This is the basis of some diabetes self-care initiatives, whereby the individual feels that an action – such as regular self-monitoring of blood glucose – is sustainable, the perceived benefits motivating the individual. This desire for action is driven by a higher value system arising from self-generated values, or derived from a religious-based system (Myers, 2000).

Cognition is a process based on knowledge, whilst emotion is centred on motivation (Bradley and Lang, 2000). For social functioning, knowledge and motivation are necessary, although intention and activation is not typical, depending on the individual's age and situation. Smyth and Arigo (2009) suggest that the attainment of new life skills and adaptation to use them requires both emotion and cognition. This is perhaps because emotions consist of energy. Emotional drive enables rapid adaptation to situational demands, helping the individual prioritise events, influencing, directing, and maintaining the behaviors necessary for dealing with these events (Chew, et al., 2014).

The stress response

If an individual becomes angry, every biological system synchronises so that the situation can be dealt with efficiently while blocking all other signals and events. When a stressful situation arises, the thalamus – relay station – signals the brainstem to prepare all major organs and muscles for fight or flight. The adrenal glands release the stress hormone cortisol to suppress the immune system, reducing inflammation if any injury is sustained in a fight. Cortisol also stimulates the brain's amygdala – responsible for generating negative emotions – to keep vigilant, producing more cortisol. This then supresses memory so only the hippocampus can recall information about how the individual reacted during a similar experience. During a stressful situation, cortisol also halts digestion and the urge to procreate, prioritising the situation at hand.

The stress response causes the release of epinephrine to speed up the heart, increasing blood supply; the pupils also dilate to allow the individual to be fully aware of any threats, such as physical attack, especially if it is dark. If the event is not a life and death situation these stress hormones act to kill off neurons in the hippocampus – the part of the brain responsible for securing memory – causing permanent memory loss. These chemical imbalances reduce immune system function and impair the release of serotonin, making the individual feel listless and depressed. If these hormonal levels continue to be elevated, this can trigger heart disease, hardening of the arteries, Type 2 diabetes, and certain types of cancer (Wax, 2013).

Emotional reactions are designed to conserve energy and rally resources to meet a specific short-term goal, meaning that emotions such as anger are usually short-lived. When emotional intensity is goal-driven, this intensity is similar to goal-driven motivation and both states are influenced by the importance of the goal. This can be seen, for example, when something interferes with the expression of anger and the emotion becomes intensified.

Rapidly altering emotions over a short time span affects health adversely, especially the cardiovascular system because of variations in blood pressure and pulse rate (Bishop, et al., 2001). An unstable emotional state can also severely upset autonomic nervous system function and pituitary/adrenal gland influence on the immune and metabolic systems (Segerstrom and Miller, 2004). Conversely, marked fluctuations in blood glucose levels are responsible for anger, depression, and anxiety with steeper glucose peaks increasing anxiety, significantly affecting health-related quality of life (Penckofer, et al., 2012).

Cognitive reappraisal and regulating emotions

Negative emotions dramatically affect health because of their effect on cognition and making short-term decisions rather than rationalised long-term choices (Worthy, et al., 2014). When the individual is consciously aware of their cognitions and alters them accordingly – with cognitive reappraisal and expressive suppression – this results in improved mental health and general wellbeing (Hu, et al., 2014).

Similar to cognitive reappraisal, the practice of mindfulness encourages the individual to concentrate on the present and be aware of their breathing and what they can see, smell, feel, and hear rather than going through life on auto-pilot; this technique can also be used to focus on pain to reduce the discomfort. Research suggests that rather than fully concentrating on a task or action, the brain wanders for around 50 percent of the day, typically lost in negative thoughts of past events, what might have happened differently, or what has already occurred (Wax, 2013).

The medial frontal cortex is a specific mind-wandering area of the brain that focusses on the self. If mindfulness is regularly practiced, the anterior cingulated cortex of the brain becomes denser – this area is responsible for attention, self-awareness and regulation, and assessing expected conflicts such as when a long-term goal might be reached. Awareness of anger, and labelling it as such is known to reduce the emotion and calm the amygdala area of the brain so that it generates fewer negative emotions. Mindfulness also activates the 'rest and digest' area of the brain, helping to regulate emotions (Wax, 2013).

Over time, the use of focused mindfulness techniques has been shown to improve mental health by changing the way the individual thinks, re-shaping the neurons of the brain – neuroplasticity. Neurons are capable of changing their pathways throughout the individual's lifetime as a result of their experiences and how they think about them; mindfulness can therefore be used to overcome harmful behaviours and thought patterns. Thoughts affect the physiology of the brain and, in a feedback loop, this physiology affects thought patterns. The brain directs negative information faster than it does positive (Wax, 2013), meaning that a bad experience is registered for future reference by the hippocampus – responsible for consolidating memory. This primes the individual for avoidance and fear, but if these emotions are directed inwardly, it can manifest as debilitation and depression (Wax, 2013). This means the individual can be the creator of his or her own stress without any external influence.

Mindfulness-based cognitive therapy – MBCT – suggests that depression should not be suppressed. This technique encourages the individual to identify where their feelings and emotions originate in order to lower the intensity. Even when mindfulness has only been practised for a few days the individual experiences reduced amygdala activity and feelings of fear, ultimately resulting physically in a steady heartbeat and normal blood pressure levels.

The individual's perception of their diabetes

The individual's health perception is a sum of health beliefs and cognitive and emotional representations or understandings. Health behaviours and clinical outcomes, such as treatment concordance, have been associated with these perceptions (Chew, et al., 2014). Perceptions are also formed about an illness based on how prolonged it is; whether the individual feels they are able to take action to improve the illness; how well the treatment works; understanding of the condition; and the direct and indirect emotional consequences experienced – symptoms and worry. In terms of Type 1 diabetes the individual's perception of coping with a condition that has no cure is constantly changing with duration of the disease, especially if Type 1 diabetes is very brittle – difficult to manage—and complications have developed.

'When Type 1 was first diagnosed I just did my injections and forgot about it. I didn't feel my diabetes was particularly serious or intrusive, and I wasn't upset or emotional about the diagnosis. I developed diabetes-related sight problems a few years later, and that's what upset me. I cried with frustration, but still didn't regard my diabetes as any kind of threat. When I'd had it for two decades, I met my husband and he encouraged me to take my diabetes seriously. I learned why I'd got sight problems and, by that time, neuropathy. I recognised that I had a serious condition and now manage it as well as possible'.

McSharry, et al., (2011) showed that perceptions following a duration of diabetes and understanding of the condition are associated with HbA1c level. Individuals with long-standing diabetes are more likely to adopt self-management behaviours such as regular foot care and blood glucose monitoring when they perceive the risk of – or already have – complications (Gale, et al., 2008). Satisfaction with health consultations and provision has been associated with the individual's illness perception and heath beliefs about their condition. Having information, education and support needs met is significantly associated with diabetes care provision satisfaction (Wilson, 2003a).

'I recently asked my diabetes nurse about improving blood glucose levels with insulin pump therapy [to tailor insulin dosages to need, rather than having two injections a day]. She was so helpful, giving me leaflets about the treatment and explaining how pump therapy might help me'.

Conversely, misconceptions about an illness can impede efforts by healthcare professionals to assist the individual's understanding of their condition (Donkin, et al., 2006), hindering self-management efforts. Individuals with Type 2 diabetes may hold a number of beliefs and misunderstandings about foot complications 'that differed somewhat from medical evidence' (Gale, et al., 2008). By ignoring medical advice and adopting poor self-care behaviours, these beliefs could potentially increase the risk of skin ulceration.

> 'I was told not to walk around the house without shoes to protect my feet from injury, but I walk barefoot or just in slippers because it's a hassle to have to keep putting shoes on'.
>
> 'If I contacted my diabetes team every time I had foot pain or hard skin, I'd never be off the phone. I don't have a podiatrist and I try-to remove the hard skin myself'.

Approximately 15 percent of people with diabetes develop a foot ulcer at some time in their life: 17 percent of ulcers result in minor or major amputation; there is a 5-year mortality rate of more than 50 percent for individuals with foot ulcers and 80 percent in those who have a diabetes-related amputation, six percent being hospitalised due to infection (Ismail, et al., 2007; Pound, et al., 2005). Gale, et al. (2008) reported that those with diabetes neglect a number of foot care behaviours, such as not reporting an injury, pain or areas of hard skin to their diabetes or foot care provider; failing to carry out daily foot checks for injury, or keeping the feet well protected. The need for self-care and prevention is therefore significant.

Diabetes distress

Positive and negative emotions impact on health outcomes, especially in the management of diabetes. Any negativity impacts both behaviourally and biologically to encourage inflammatory changes which characterise diabetes mellitus (Misra, et al., 2012; Sarwar, et al., 2010).

Negative emotions can also amplify many health risks such as heart disease and depression. Stress, anxiety and depression in turn are related to compromised immune and inflammation responses which are known to exacerbate conditions associated with ageing, such as cardiovascular diseases; osteoporosis; arthritis; Alzheimer's disease; frailty and functional decline; Type 1 and Type 2 diabetes; certain cancers, and tooth and gum disease.

In addition, negative emotions affecting the body's immune response, contribute to prolonged infections, adversely affecting glycaemic control and delaying wound healing, particularly for those with diabetes and poor circulation. The association between emotional distress and

inflammatory responses is likely to result in a vicious cycle, where negativity contributes to or causes the health issue and consequently, the
condition exacerbates further negative emotions.

Diabetes distress describes the emotional distress resulting from living
with diabetes and the necessity of relentless self-management; heightened distress affects one in four people with Type 2 diabetes treated
with insulin and one in six people with Type 2 who are not insulin
treated (Diabetes UK, 2019). Increased distress accompanies poorly
managed blood glucose levels due to their effect on brain chemistry,
although diabetes distress may still be seen with good diabetes self-
management and optimal HbA1c levels. Diabetes distress is more
common than diabetes-related depression, and may be misdiagnosed as
such as symptoms are similar, therefore, distress is managed in a diabetes
care context (Diabetes UK, 2019).

Coping mechanisms

It has been suggested that 'future-orientated thinking' or 'proactive
coping' is necessary for individuals to assimilate a desired health behaviour (Aspinwall and Tedeschi, 2010). This suggestion does not acknowledge that the individual must want to cope with their ill health,
rather than the healthcare professional alone; there must be proactivity
and recognition of the benefit of their actions. When future thinking/
proactive coping is practised, the individual continually expects adverse
outcomes if the desired behaviour is not continued – such as the difficulty of sticking to a diabetes diet when on holiday. This then becomes a
stressful situation because the individual wants to stick to their diet, but
temptation or differences in available foods make this more difficult.

By exercising proactive coping, the individual plans a way to overcome
this barrier – perhaps self-catering on holiday, for example – reinforcing
the strategy to keep their goal possible. In a study of newly-diagnosed
Type 1 diabetes, Thoolen, et al. (2009) found that proactive individuals
were better able to maintain a long-term – at one year – regime of diabetic
diet and physical activity than those who exhibited self-efficacy behaviour
or articulated a plan to do so.

Proactivity instead of future-orientated thinking has been shown to be
more easily achieved when applied to health behaviour (Chew, et al.,
2014). However, depending on the impact of diabetes and its complications, the individual may require a high degree of support from
healthcare professionals and family members in order to achieve any self-
management proactivity. Gervey, et al. (2005) suggest this is how the
individual gains the cognitive and emotional ability to succeed.

Conversely, individuals with the necessary cognitive and emotional support put this into practice and feel able to succeed. Therefore, proactive diabetes self-management is readily undertaken so the individual copes well with their condition with the correct illness perception, seeing its position in their life, with self-efficacy and the ability to self-regulate (Chew, et al., 2014).

A future with diabetes may be overwhelming, especially if there is poor glycaemic control and/or chronic complications, making coping with present self-management demands difficult. One of the greatest challenges of diabetes management is controlling fluctuations in blood glucose levels. As we have seen, this requires a high level of motivation, persistence, attentiveness and expectation by the individual, plus the expert knowledge of the diabetes specialist. Common causes of worsening blood glucose control include infections, stress, depression, and certain medications. Therefore, both the individual and their consultant should be aware of measures to regain control when glucose rises sharply.

'My [Type 1] diabetes control is erratic and I've had problems managing it. My consultant tried everything, from testing for coeliac disease to testing for delayed stomach emptying, but found nothing wrong. I then basically stopped trying hard to control my diabetes because I couldn't cope with the enormity of it all'.

'When I had my COVID vaccinations, my blood sugar shot up and stayed there each time, no matter what I did. I didn't have an infection, and the problem lasted for about a month. This was made worse when I saw my GP and diabetes consultant, as they kept reminding me that future complications were looming. It was like scare tactics but, instead of helping, I was being blamed. I had no options and I didn't get any help. Everything calmed down on its own in the end – I assume it was a reaction to the vaccine'.

'I don't want to think about my diabetes in twenty years' time – just too depressing'.

These views show that coping behaviour is unique to the individual: some have overwhelming diabetes problems, so coping may not match up to the expected goals that healthcare professionals would assume gives the individual the best possible quality of life.

Diabetes control can fluctuate in severity, making it harder for the individual to cope at these times. An event such as severe hyperglycemia and associated diabetic ketoacidosis – DKA – is a medical emergency. DKA occurs when there is prolonged hyperglycaemia causing the body to break down fats as an alternative source of energy to the glucose that cannot be used when there is a lack of insulin, resulting in acid by-products. Such emergencies can be prevented with effective self-management of hyperglycaemia.

Racial/ethnic differences in diabetes and its complications

It is well-documented that racial/ethnic minorities experience a higher prevalence of diabetes than non-minority individuals (Golden, et al., 2012). Multiple factors contribute to these inequalities, such as biological and clinical features, as well as health system and social influences. Physical inactivity and smoking – a coping mechanism – are well-recognised risk factors for developing Type 2 diabetes; research has shown that race/ethnicity predicts reduced levels of physical activity (Kurian and Cardarelli, 2007) and increased smoking behaviour (WHO, 2021). Higher smoking rates among racial/ethnic minorities may explain the higher prevalence of diabetes and peripheral arterial disease in this population.

Abnormally elevated blood glucose levels over time trigger the onset of diabetic complications, making self-monitoring of blood glucose (SMBG) a key behaviour in diabetes self-management. There is no evidence of racial/ethnic differences associated with SMBG behaviour; some studies have suggested non-concordance for certain populations, although alternative research has shown this not to be the case (Golden, et al., 2012; Kirk, et al., 2007).

A causal factor of hyperglycaemia and poorly-managed diabetes is depression: depression is a well-known comorbidity of diabetes, while hyperglycaemia in diabetes adversely affects mental health, triggering depression. Depression impairs diabetes self-care behaviours and ethnic minorities have a greater prevalence of depression; depression is also more likely to remain undiagnosed and untreated (Wagner, et al., 2007). A lower level of concordance with following medication advice and taking up screening invitations has also been reported concerning minority populations, leading to worsening severity of diabetes symptoms prior to diagnosis (Karter, et al., 2007). Barriers to healthcare for ethnic minorities therefore exist in a number of areas, not least potential language barriers impeding the communication process between healthcare professional and patient; there may be difficulties in the patient understanding or hearing correctly a foreign accent, and vice-versa.

While English is the primary language of over 90 percent of UK residents (Gov UK, 2019) 138,000 people living in the UK do not speak English at all and over 60 percent of these are women. It is also important to recognise that an understanding of medical terminology should not be assumed by English and non-English speakers. Language barriers can impede communication and impact on the quality and uptake of care, including physical and mental health outcomes (Berry, 2016; Misra-Hebert and Isaacson, 2012; Furler and Kokanovic, 2010). Healthcare professionals must therefore adapt their communications to meet patient need, involving the use of the patient's family, friends and interpreters to ensure the message is received.

Diabetes self-management

As we have seen, effective diabetes self-management requires the implementation of positive behaviours and suppression of undesirable, competing behaviours (Bandura, 1991). Self-regulation involves influences such as self-discipline, self-reactive influences and self-gratification – satisfaction – to carry out a desired behaviour. The behaviour must be perceived as valuable – for example, regular blood glucose self-monitoring, in order for it to generate the necessary motivation to continue that behaviour. When there is proactive consideration of the new behaviour and its effects, or it gains approval from others, such as the diabetes nurse, this encourages continuation. According to Bandura (1991), the individual may compare the outcome of a behaviour – for example, reducing HbA1c level – to previous personal or social achievements. This comparison allows significance to be associated with the behaviour, enabling further self-evaluation. Through this repeated process, skills are acquired so the individual develops a sense of self-efficacy (Bandura, 1977b).

The adverse outcome of self-regulation suggests that the individual could become overly pleased with their achievements and conceited with 'self-praise' or, conversely, dysfunctional due to misconception, misjudgments of 'self' and prone to depression and destructive behaviours (Chew, et al., 2014; Bandura, 2001). This mechanism of acquiring a sense of self-regulatory behaviour may put the individual's 'internal standards' at odds with 'universal moral standards', thus leading to helplessness and hopelessness (Bandura, 1999a; 1999b). This is probable for individuals with diabetes who – despite proactive self-care – may not achieve the desired results.

Successful diabetes self-management

It is believed that a positive outlook towards self-management of diabetes, resilience and a sense of wellbeing can be gained from the external support of family, friends, healthcare professionals and others with the same condition. Positive diabetes self-care behaviours and health-related quality of life are strongly associated with positive mental health (Chan, et al., 2009). Several studies show that positive emotional health – resilience, wellbeing, gratitude and influence – are strongly associated with treatment concordance, exercise and frequent self-monitoring of blood glucose, leading to improved health outcomes – specifically HbA1c, health status, health-related quality of life, and reduced mortality risk (Jaser, et al., 2014; Robertson, et al., 2013). Despite this, the impact of positive emotional health has been investigated to a lesser degree.

Similarly, little research has examined the effect of positive mental health on blood glucose levels (Skaff, et al., 2009; Ryff, et al., 2006). Available studies have focused on poor glycaemic control, depressive symptoms and the subsequent negative effect on HbA1c levels (Aitkens, 2012; Fisher, et al., 2010). Learning to value positive perceptions, intuition and reasoning and increasing levels of motivation to embrace a positive lifestyle will ultimately affect diabetes self-management, decision making and quality of life outcomes. This is undoubtedly due to the positive effect of optimistic emotions on the endocrine and immune systems which are undermined in diabetes (Jaremka, et al., 2013). This ultimately encourages self-efficacy, positive behaviours, resilience and health-related quality of life, which feeds back into the loop of improved immune and endocrine function.

Self-efficacy applied to diabetes self-care

Self-efficacy is considered as a predisposing factor that can be deteriorated in chronic conditions like diabetes; efficacy in life is increased by strategic thought. Self-efficacy is the individual's belief that they can achieve effective diabetes self-management. This concept is based on self-regulation and is achieved through the motivation for self-monitoring, goal-setting and evaluation behaviours which are carried out despite any encountered barriers. Therefore, following a diabetes diagnosis, the individual's belief in their own ability may motivate them to make particular health choices and persevere when difficulties arise.

Behaviour change can be achieved by changing the way a person thinks. Self-efficacy describes the individual's confidence to carry out a specific positive health behaviour. Dixon (2008) suggested that an individual's self-efficacy may be significantly reduced if they fear the consequences of trying something new; if they have previous experience of failure – for example, smoking cessation; or if their emotional/mental state poses barriers such as depression and anxiety. Self-efficacy is a good predictor of behaviour change and improved psychological outcomes.

Prior research has shown that improving diabetes self-efficacy can improve self-management behavior, although little is known about the applicability of this research across race/ethnicity and health literacy levels. Sakar, et al., (2006) examined the relationship between diabetes self-efficacy and self-management behavior in an urban, diverse, low-income population with a high prevalence of limited health literacy. Patients were more likely to report optimal diet, exercise, self-monitoring of blood glucose, and foot care, but not medication concordance. The associations between self-efficacy and self-management were consistent across race/ethnicity and health literacy levels.

Self-efficacy and motivation underpin intention to undertake a specific behaviour, whether it be giving up smoking or increasing the frequency of SMBG and acting on the results to self-manage diabetes more effectively. Self-efficacy also enables the achievement of goals; once an action is decided upon, self-efficacy helps maintain the effort required to overcome any barriers to sustaining that behaviour. It has been suggested that intention to undertake a behaviour is different to planning, initiating or maintaining that behaviour (Sniehotta, et al., 2005), showing that self-efficacy is important at all stages of behavioural change (Wilson, 2009; West, 2006).

'I use a continuous glucose sensor with my insulin pump because of frequent hypoglycaemia, often becoming unconscious during the night. My diabetes consultant arranged funding for the necessary technology, the nurse explained how to use it, and I set about learning how it worked. When I tried to insert the glucose sensor into my abdomen at home, I had problems so, after several attempts, I gave up. A few weeks later I tried again and it worked, showing my ongoing glucose levels. The thought of how the technology could help me avoid severe hypos motivated me to carry on until I succeeded with getting the glucose monitoring system to work'.

The self-efficacy for this individual to master their diabetes self-management technology arises from learned capability. This is gained via experience where effort is required to adopt the behaviour (Bandura, 1977a). By using varying experiences and by processing efficacy information, learned capability and confidence result. Bandura (1997b) also suggested that an expectation of efficacy is made real by the addition of motivating thoughts, values and beliefs which carry the behaviour towards completion. If the individual is unable to make beneficial health decisions due to – for example – depression, wellbeing is affected as self-regulation and self-efficacy rely on proactivity and independent judgement.

There are seven essential self-care behaviours that predict good diabetes outcomes:

- Healthy eating
- Being physically active
- Regular self-monitoring of blood glucose
- Concordance with advised medications
- Good problem-solving skills
- Healthy coping skills
- Risk reduction behaviour

Self-determination

Once an intention is decided, self-determination acts to change that intention into a real behaviour (Baumeister and Tierney, 2012). Similar to willpower, self-determination requires effort and perseverance to make an appropriate choice when/if an adverse impulse is faced. Self-determination defers the need for short-term gratification in favour of receiving a long-term return (Duckworth, 2011), such as sticking to a diabetic diet in order to maintain good glycaemic control. Thus, the individual overcomes emotional urges with cognitive reasoning. Chew, et al. (2014) described the force of self-determination as 'an educated spirit that grows in understanding and has the ability to control emotions'. Willpower has also been described as a trait seen in young children which remains into adulthood (Hagger, 2013; Moffitt, et al., 2011).

Self-determination is associated with increased academic ability in school-age children, greater self-esteem, reduced rates of substance abuse, greater financial security and better mental and physical health (Hagger, 2013). However, this influence is reduced if self-determination is repeated in a short space of time, resulting in poor self-control when the next immediate challenge is faced (Baumeister, 2003). The individual may want to address several negative behaviours – such as over-eating, smoking, substance abuse – being unsuccessful in their attempts due to 'willpower failure' (Tsukayama, et al., 2010; Vohs and Faber, 2007). As such, self-determination/willpower is stronger and more effective when the focus is on just one goal rather than multiple aims (Webb and Sheeran, 2003), for example, incorporating regular exercise into a lifestyle with diabetes. Motivated individuals who have a positive mood, attitude and beliefs are less likely to have low self-determination and are more likely to see it sustained (Vohs, et al., 2011; Muraven, et al., 2008). It can be seen that positive emotions boost self-determination/willpower, and negative emotions may be suppressed by self-determination when consciously applied to the situation.

Resilience

Resilience is defined as the ability to maintain psychological and physical wellbeing when faced with adverse life events by drawing on self-esteem, self-efficacy, self-mastery and optimism (Rutter, 2012; Yi-Frazier, et al., 2010). These qualities are especially beneficial when applied to diabetes self-management. Depending on the individual's personality, difficult life events are perceived as either stressful, threatening or challenging (Steinhardt, et al., 2009). Resilience for the elderly individual with Type 2 diabetes enables successful social functioning (Mertens, et al., 2012), suggesting that self-reliance is more beneficial to mental health than reliance on others. Resilience has also been likened to willpower because, with regular application, it increases over time (Muraven, et al., 1999). Thus, a focus on wellbeing and resilience is beneficial. An example of diabetes-related resilience is shown below.

'I was given a date for steroid injections into my lower back. When I arrived at the hospital, I was told this wouldn't be going ahead – it had been decided (by a healthcare professional who had never even met me) that I was too high risk for the procedure as I had Type 1 diabetes. I was really surprised by my reaction – I was disappointed and felt like I'd been wrongly judged and discriminated against, but I wasn't angry, upset or depressed. I was stoical and just took it in my stride. If this had happened 20 years ago, I would have reacted very negatively, becoming depressed and anxious; I contacted the Head of the hospital, explained why their decision was wrong – he apologised profusely for that member of staff's decision and arranged for the steroid injections to take place'.

It is clear that health-related adversity 'breeds resilience' so it is not surprising that individuals with diabetes are well-practised at calling on this resource. Experience gained in diabetes self-management over the duration of the condition enables the individual to become strong in this respect, described as the 'steeling effect' (Rutter, 2013; Bradshaw, et al., 2007a) whereby strong layers of resilience are built up. Because this is outwardly visible, it is possible for healthcare professionals to objectively view an individual's resilience to a health-related event – such as the diagnosis of diabetes or a complication – and to assess coping ability and impact. In this way, healthcare professionals do not have to rely on subjective assessment of the individual's feelings.

Resilience must be drawn from the individual's resources and reserves, formed from internal strength when faced with difficulty – shown externally as hope, fortitude, optimism, happiness and vitality. This comes from the individual's values and beliefs, shaped by emotional learning, knowledge or religious beliefs (Steinhardt, et al., 2009; Bradshaw, et al., 2007b). A lack of resilience – especially in those with diabetes – therefore manifests as depression, with the individual feeling overwhelmed, disgruntled, apathetic or guilty. Individual resources to deal with adverse events are gained from the individual's external support network, such as family, friends, and support groups. Thus, reserves are key to resilience as they involve more personal qualities when faced with adversity. This is because adversity is felt at a personal level, demanding a personal response (Chew, et al., 2014). However, Myers (2000) suggests that self-reliance can lead to self-delusion.

Positive diabetes management interventions

A review of current literature suggests that there is an absence of positive health intervention programmes for those with diabetes in the UK. Much literature cites the need for mental health support, but does not detail the provision. Psychological intervention to enhance positive health needs to be person-centred rather than a non-specific programme attended by a group with either Type 1 or Type 2 diabetes. There is no doubt that diabetes also takes its toll socially, and these issues have been highlighted as important determinants of self-care (Clark and Utz, 2014). Wilson (2003) showed there was a lack of psychosocial support for individuals, the majority of diabetes clinics having no trained psychologist or counsellor as part of the diabetes team. In 2021, an internet search of the services offered by diabetes clinics across the UK showed a similar picture, suggesting that little has changed.

Key messages in this chapter:

- As many as 50 percent of individuals being diagnosed with diabetes already have a feeling of adverse psychological wellbeing.
- Having either Type 1 or Type 2 diabetes can impact adversely on the individual and their life, not just with regard to disease self-management.
- The National Service Framework priorities for diabetes care document states that, 'all individuals with diabetes should be provided with educational and psychological support, with the aim of facilitating and supporting self-management'.
- Positive and negative emotions have a huge impact on health outcomes, especially in the management of diabetes. Negativity impacts both behaviourally and biologically to encourage inflammatory changes which characterise diabetes mellitus.
- Positive emotional health in terms of resilience, wellbeing, gratitude and influence are strongly associated with treatment concordance, exercise and frequent SMBG, leading to improved health outcomes – specifically HbA1c, health status, health-related quality of life, and reduced mortality risk.
- Proactivity instead of future-orientated thinking is more easily achieved by the individual when applied to health behaviour.
- All of the most common mental health disorders – such as depression, anxiety, phobias, seasonal affective disorder, eating disorders and obsessive-compulsive disorder – can interfere with diabetes management.
- Psychological intervention to enhance positive health must be person-centred rather than a non-specific programme attended by a group of patients with either Type 1 or Type 2 diabetes.

2 Diabetes and Psychosocial Issues

Psychological issues – emotional and mental health concerns—such as diabetes distress and depression, are frequently experienced by adults with diabetes and are associated with poor self-management, diabetes complications, reduced quality of life, and increased health care costs. In 2001, the Diabetes Attitudes, Wishes and Needs (DAWN) study (Peyrot, et al., 2005; 2013) showed that self-management of diabetes was considered poor by those with the condition and the health professionals who delivered their care. Wilson (2003) and Alberti (2002) have reported low recognition and understanding by healthcare professionals of emotional issues and diabetes-specific distress. There is a focus on psychological wellbeing for people with diabetes. However, due to NHS resource limitations in recent years, interdisciplinary diabetes care involving a clinical psychologist or counsellor is uncommon. Without specialist funding, it is impossible to integrate psychological support into diabetes care, provide screening for anxiety and depression, or impart psycho-educational resources to those with diabetes.

Psychosocial issues for people with diabetes

It could be said that altered metabolic parameters in diabetes make it difficult – if not practically impossible – to rectify this imbalance, so the condition can never be fully controlled to achieve normal blood glucose levels.

Concordance

Concordance refers to the extent that the individual follows a given medical treatment regime; non-concordance describes failure to follow the advice of healthcare professionals. Rather than being blamed or

DOI: 10.4324/9781003260219-3

judged, this can be considered as reasoned decision-making if the individual does not follow health recommendations.

Although empowerment – informed choice – supports concordance and does not associate non-concordance with failure to follow a diabetes self-management regime, the individual may be unable to fully concur with medical advice. This view has been described as rational decision-making by Vahdat, et al. (2014) and Day (1995), where medical regime guidance may be ignored in the belief that this will improve quality of life. Individuals with diabetes are faced with a number of behavioural choices, including concordance with some but not all expected behaviours; this is underpinned by personal health beliefs and may involve a simple refusal to manage a complex and chronic medical condition (Donnovan, et al., 2002; Horne, 1997).

It is difficult to measure the level to which diabetes health advice is followed because this often relies on self-assessment and self-reporting. Despite this, engagement in certain health behaviours can be determined by other means (Pouwer, et al., 2003). The frequency of prescription requests for blood glucose test strips, and the results of HbA1c blood glucose measurements – the amount of glucose sticking to the red blood cells over a 3-month period – can be correlated with the reported self-management behaviour. However, a poor relationship exists between concordance with different health behaviours, such as monitoring glucose levels, following dietary recommendations, taking regular exercise, and taking the correct amount of medication at the right time. This means that some aspects of diabetes self-management are undertaken more readily than others and this is common for all health behaviours; the National Collaboration Centre for Primary Care (2008) found that almost 50 percent of patients forgot to take prescribed medication.

Concordance is a behaviour that does not remain the same over time; it has been shown to increase in accordance with duration of diabetes (Settineri, et al., 2019). Connor and Norman (2015) suggested that some unsuitable diabetes health behaviours are sustained due to a lack of support for changing that behaviour. Non-concordance is a major barrier to the acceptance of diabetes treatments such as multiple daily insulin injections or insulin pump therapy because they require a high level of attentiveness and motivation to use them effectively. These treatments are often the only way to improve glycaemic control, but the individual must adopt an intensive diabetes regime and be proactive in their diabetes self-care: they must want and be enabled to improve glycaemic control to prevent or delay long-term complications of diabetes, such as eye and kidney disease.

The Diabetes Control and Complications Trial (DCCT, 1993) for Type 1 diabetes, and the UK Prospective Diabetes Study (UKPDS, 1998a, UKPDS, 1998b) for Type 2 diabetes, showed that intensive diabetes self-management using either multiple daily injections or insulin pump therapy is essential in reducing the risk of micro- and macro-vascular complications – small and large blood vessel disease which can lead to stroke and heart disease. If the individual is unable or unwilling to engage fully in intensive diabetes self-management, these treatment options become ineffective.

Having an understanding of the consequences of poor glycaemic control and the skills and motivation to assess potential health risks is not the same as effective self-management of diabetes. In the same way, access to diabetes education does not automatically increase knowledge, or encourage self-care and self-management behaviour towards con-cordance with medical advice – the distinction between attitude change and behaviour change means that one does not equal the other. As a result, a change must occur in both the individual's attitude and beha-viour so that diabetes is managed for the right reasons. This, though, is easier said than done when considering issues such as acceptance of the condition, health beliefs, social situation, depression, incapacity, or a combination of these factors resulting in poor health outcomes which are inextricably linked and beyond the individual's control.

Locus of control

Locus of control refers to an individual's perception about the underlying main causes of events in his/her life. This is a term applied to a 'personality difference' which influences the perception of a stressful event and its im-pact on subsequent behaviour. The individual's locus of control is the de-gree of perceived control over a situation or event – therefore an individual with a high degree of control over a situation is less likely to become stressed by it. This level of control is termed an internal locus because the individual has control over their environment and they can direct their life to some degree. The locus of control is crucial in determining a good or bad re-lationship between patient and healthcare provider; a major determinant of stress and emotion is perception of ability to control a situation. A perceived lack of control over life events – lives dictated by, or subject to the actions of others – have an external locus of control.

Thus, stress is far more significant in the lives of those with an external locus and this may be unhealthy when accompanied by perceived powerlessness in a stressful situation. This state of mind was termed 'learned helplessness' by Seligman (1975), who also attributed some forms of depression to feeling helpless. Burns (2001) suggests that this occurs when the individual finds that they are in a situation where their responses are irrelevant to that situation, when there is no correct response, or where inappropriate responses have been learned. When this behaviour is applied to different situations over time, the individual believes they are unable to cope with the world. Seligman suggested that this can be overcome with the provision of positive encouragement to achieve in small tasks, gradually progressing to more complex ones.

When applied to diabetes, the loss of control over health may result in an inability to manage the condition successfully, especially if the individual has brittle Type 1 diabetes. Learning occurs from successful past experience if this success was based on skill and not luck. It is also the case that the individual copes better with stress if they perceive they have some control over any outcome concerning diabetes management. A belief that nothing can be done about having a chronic health condition demanding ongoing self-management often leads to depression, anxiety and anger due to loss of initiative. It is therefore important for diabetes healthcare professionals to recognise these emotive issues, offering support for the achievement of small steps to increase confidence to escape a situation of learned helplessness.

Motivation and health beliefs

Motivation has been defined in psychological terms as internal processes that spur us on to satisfy some need (Burns, 2001; Sheldon, et al., 2000). It has also been explained more simply as the reason for action. There are multiple factors associated with carrying out an action and numerous opinions have been suggested concerning how motivation operates. Many emphasise goal-setting and conscious decision-making as a reason for carrying out health behaviours, although negative emotions also drive growth.

Probably the best-known theory of motivation in human behaviour is Maslow's (1943) Hierarchy of Needs model, explaining the acquisition of knowledge and understanding – with emphasis on the role of the individual in achieving their own physical, social and cultural needs – as a path to knowledge. The individual's needs in this model are stacked by order of importance in a pyramid with psychological needs forming the broad base. As the pyramid rises, safety needs come next, followed by love and belonging, self-esteem, self-actualisation, and finally the intellectual needs of understanding and knowledge. Evidence-based PhD. research examining motivation for self-management in Type 2 diabetes found that life values were critical motivational factors for engaging in diabetes self-management (Oftedal, 2011). The results also suggested that goals related to self-management were formulated in more general than specific terms.

For those with diabetes, Maslow's theory implies that healthcare professionals will be unable to impart appropriate knowledge to an individual if emotional needs are not addressed first. Because motivation is necessary to achieve a reachable goal, motivation for diabetes self-care is driven by success, creating a cyclical process: motivation enables the behaviour, while the success of that behaviour creates the motivation for repetition – self-efficacy. As previously mentioned, empowerment has been cited as the key to this process in diabetes self-management through knowledge, control, and the ability to implement decisions.

Motivation can be internal or external, explaining the desire an individual has to undertake certain health behaviours without receiving an immediate reward – this motivation arises from satisfaction with feeling proficient and self-determined. Conscious and sub-conscious factors therefore influence motivation, along with internal and external drives; personal beliefs about the consequences of an action, the perceived outcome of any change in behaviour, and the attitudes and approval of others. Motivation is a core principle of the COM-B model of health behaviour and a key principle of the Behaviour Change Wheel, applied specifically to the degree of motivation an individual has for diabetes self-care.

The individual bases their behaviour on their perception of the severity of diabetes. Therefore, the level of self-care an individual is prepared to engage in is strongly related to a belief that preventative action will reduce the threat of poor control of diabetes. As we have already seen, however, the degree of motivation for different self-care activities varies, meaning that some behaviours are undertaken more frequently than others, and this changes with the individual's circumstances. Research by Patel, et al. (2015) showed that specific health beliefs and behaviours correlate with ability to manage diabetes treatment demands – suggesting that older individuals, those with chronic complications such as sight difficulties, or those with long-duration diabetes may have impaired motivation for certain self-care activities.

In terms of health beliefs, perceived susceptibility to diabetes and its chronic complications may be both a motivating and a de-motivating factor, as well as clarifying the perceived benefits of carrying out self-care activities.

'When you've got diabetes, complications are bound to happen because your body doesn't deal with sugar normally. I've known people who've developed complications despite good diabetes control, and others who pay no attention when their sugars are often high'.

'No matter how much time and effort I invest in looking after my diabetes, I can't get good blood glucose control'.

Negative health beliefs are an obvious barrier to achieving good diabetes control and management. Although a specific health belief scale has been devised by some researchers (Gutierrez and Long, 2011; Bradley, 1994), problems have been encountered when trying to apply these scales to the understanding of diabetes as a chronic condition. This was especially an issue in the past when the 'compliance approach' dominated how diabetes self-care was measured, rather than the current patient-centred approach, where care is tailored to individual needs.

As health beliefs are modified by changes in behaviour, the subsequent belief is a result of the behaviour after the outcome is achieved. This may not be the same as the belief that predicted the behaviour and perhaps predicted the change. Ultimately, this outcome may cause reversion to earlier and less-healthy diabetes management behaviour, with poorer glycaemic control. Broome and Llewelyn (1995) suggested that the predictive power of the individual's health beliefs in chronic disease may be naturally limited because of this feedback loop. Additionally, in order to achieve a certain level of self-management behaviour, awareness of this is required via the provision of information, diabetes education and support.

Karim, et al. (2016) examined perceived susceptibility to predict whether young women with Type 2 diabetes would successfully adopt diabetes self-care behaviours. Health beliefs were found not to predict all aspects of self-care and self-management activity. Significant correlations were found between active self-care behaviours and self-monitoring of blood glucose, but not for other outcomes, such as exercise and diet. It is the case that there are distinct differences between the perceived benefits of health regime concordance for those with long-duration diabetes, and for older individuals. This highlights the difficulty of applying a one-size-fits-all model of behaviour to diabetes regime concordance because many variables – such as age, duration of diabetes, and chronic complications – must be accounted for in the effects.

Encouraging self-efficacy

Interventions designed to encourage self-efficacy in health behaviour are sporadic, and even fewer have been aimed specifically at diabetes self-care. Interventions based on a particular theoretical model aiming to address behaviour change impact on behaviour alone, rather than the components that make up that behaviour, such as self-efficacy or motivation. In his Social Cognitive Theory, Bandura (2000) suggested that self-efficacy can be enhanced by tackling barriers to behaviour change in manageable stages:

• Observing and learning from successful change in others that the individual regards as similar to their own circumstances;
• Possessing a positive mental attitude towards attaining success, whilst avoiding stress and negative emotions using relaxation techniques.

Interventions based on behaviour change rather than the components making up the targeted behaviour have been criticised for using varying methods – such as providing tailored information, and employing goal-setting or relapse-prevention strategies (Dixon, 2008). Because of the varying inclusion of certain concepts under the umbrella of behaviour change with poor outcomes, the Behaviour Change Wheel was developed from 19 frameworks of behaviour change to identify sources of behaviour that can be targeted by intervention (Mitchie, et al., 2014).

Focusing on changing behaviour to make a difference

In order to be specific and successful, health interventions must only target a single behaviour – such as addiction – and employ measures to overcome that behaviour. In terms of diabetes care, one-to-one health education tends to be employed as there are no specific interventions that target poor self-care behaviour. For those with Type 2 diabetes that has developed due to obesity and a sedentary lifestyle – where insulin cannot act effectively due to the presence of excess fat surrounding the body cells, interventions to target obesity may be of value. In terms of evidence-based healthcare, Dyson (2012) has suggested that individuals who receive intensive counselling regarding behavioural intention achieve a greater weight loss than those who do not.

An approach may be employed to encourage physical activity, where emphasis is placed on decreasing physical inactivity rather than increasing activity. Thus, physical activity is incorporated into lifestyle – such as taking the stairs rather than the lift – and using reminders to change behaviour via frequent contact with healthcare professionals – such as text messaging adolescents with Type 1 diabetes, prompting them to share blood glucose test results with their diabetes team. While this last approach has proved successful in encouraging improved health behaviour, it could be viewed as de-motivating if acceptable blood glucose results are not being achieved and this also relies on self-reporting of behaviour.

Awareness of a potential change to health behaviour enables adoption of the new or altered behaviour. Webb and Sheeran (2006) examined the strength of intention driving behaviour change correlated with health behaviour and its outcome; risk awareness literature; skill enhancement approaches and goal setting actions. Despite a medium to large change in intention, only a small to medium change in behaviour was achieved. As would be expected, interventions where the individual had reduced control over their situation were less successful – for example, the intention to lose weight and exercise more in Type 1 diabetes when hypoglycaemia is frequent and unexpected. This situation requires the individual to eat or drink unplanned sweet foods to increase blood glucose levels. Additionally, severe hypoglycaemia leads to intense cravings for starchy, high-carbohydrate foods as the brain tries to protect itself from a lack of glucose that it needs for fuel (Wilson, 2014).

It is clear that the main barrier to change is the individual themselves: once a change in health behaviour is firmly rooted, the process can begin (Thoolen, et al., 2009). A trigger factor such as a health scare or intervention may be the reason action is taken – but this decision must be the individual's. Behavioural change interventions on their own have little impact on health outcomes if the individual is unwilling or unready to change. Therefore, the reason a technique or intervention is successful is down to the individual's motivation and ability to change behaviour rather than the clarity of the strategy itself.

The best way to help implement effective diabetes self-management behaviours involves a multi-faceted assessment process. The individual must understand what they will gain from engaging in appropriate behaviours; this is dependent on motivation and attitude rather than knowledge and skills alone. Any theoretical framework for diabetes education must recognise the unique issues, goals, motivations and perceived barriers pertinent to each individual. Key interventions aiming to improve glycaemic control have provided guidance on the clinical management of diabetes (Diabetes Control and Complications Trial, 1993) but there is little guidance regarding how or why people are able to change.

Wilson (2009) examined whether communication with health professionals influenced behaviour change for proactive individuals with Type 1 diabetes using intensive treatments – multiple daily insulin injections (MDI) or insulin pump therapy treatment. During telephone interviews, the individuals commented on whether diabetes services had enabled effective glycaemic control and self-management; whether they had changed the way they managed their diabetes using intensive methods; what motivated change; who helped them make changes, and whether maintenance of change was difficult.

'When I was waiting to go from injections to a pump, I looked after myself more. I did more blood tests and checked carbohydrate values on food and drink… My diabetes consultant then decided that I didn't need an insulin pump because I'd improved my glucose levels with injections and better self-management. Now the opportunity for a pump has been taken away, I don't feel motivated to bother'.

'Managing diabetes is like having a demanding child: constantly testing my blood; watching what I eat; calculating insulin dosage for food eaten; when it will be working, etc. Then trying to fit all this in with everything else I have to do in my life, like work and the kids. You try hard, then the nurse or doctor tells you off for not making enough effort! It's virtually impossible.'

Contemplation, maintenance or relapse of diabetes self-management behaviours occurred for different reasons according to treatment type. For those taking MDI, motivation to improve glycaemic control was suggested by healthcare professionals to enable progression to insulin pump therapy treatment, so change was due to incentive. This is contradictory, however, because pump therapy tends to only be initiated where there is a clinical need, with inability to keep blood glucose levels stable any other way (NICE, 2003). If improved diabetes control is achievable with insulin injections and behaviour change – requiring frequent SMBG and intensive self-management – pump therapy, funded by the NHS, is an unnecessary expense.

With the means to do so, Wilson (2009) found that individuals treating their diabetes with MDI or pump therapy improved self-management behaviours, enabled by primary care health professionals and the flexibility offered by these intensive diabetes treatment methods.

'I think my GP assumes I know more about my diabetes than I actually do, but he makes me feel confident in discussing changes to my diet and management regime. I always go to him if I need any help with my diabetes, rather than my consultant, who I only see once a year'.

'I wanted to improve my blood sugar results so I physically felt better. I discussed this with my diabetes nurse at my annual check-up, and she helped me do this with some good suggestions and support'.

Insulin pump users have already adopted a treatment change, maintaining intensive management behaviour due to the benefits of improved glycaemic control and a reduction in long-term complications of diabetes. Insulin pump use is like an artificial pancreas and insulin can be administered as and when necessary in very small doses to achieve a more physiological insulin delivery.

'I need to have a little bit of insulin even if I'm exercising because the liver releases glucose to the muscles which can put blood sugar levels up. I can do this easily with an insulin pump but giving a small dose of insulin was never easy or accurate with an insulin syringe or pen. I also now test my blood glucose before exercising to make sure I'm not too low or too high, as this can put a strain on the heart. I now feel confident to exercise regularly and enjoy it without worry'.

Pump therapy enables proactive diabetes self-management behaviour, preventing or delaying the worsening of existing chronic complications of diabetes. The level of perceived self-efficacy is high among those managing their diabetes with insulin pump therapy because they want to be masters of their diabetes self-management.

'I have some retinopathy and, since using pump therapy to treat my diabetes intensively, this has remained stable for 13 years now. Because retinopathy is the leading cause of blindness in people with diabetes, this motivates me to continue using a pump and doing frequent blood glucose tests'.

'I've mastered pump therapy because it's a technology that helps me have control over Type 1 diabetes, rather than it having control over me'.

Intensive self-management of diabetes using MDI or pump therapy requires proactivity and motivation to utilise the treatment and prevent, reduce, or stabilise chronic complications. This requires tailored advice and support from healthcare professionals to achieve and maintain effective diabetes self-management. The previous examples from individuals adopting intensive diabetes self-management methods show that the individual must be ready for change and ultimately must also want to change their behaviour.

However, an individual may contemplate and plan behaviour change – with or without an intervention – but be unable to take this further. The perceived demands of acting on frequent blood tests and maintaining the motivation to inject insulin multiple times a day at the correct times and in the correct dosages to achieve good control of blood glucose requires a high level of motivation, ability and determination.

Motivation for diabetes self-care relies on perceived vulnerability to complications and a high degree of self-efficacy. Health information may trigger the desire to improve diabetes control – even if no complications of diabetes are apparent – due to health beliefs and the awareness of a perceived threat to current or future health: the individual must want to change and be ready for change. Many individuals with diabetes often do not engage in appropriate self-care behaviours because they are not ready for change, aware that they need to change, or because they have not been triggered into making a change.

Adopting intensive self-management behaviour to prevent complications has not been shown in the wider diabetes population. What is important is a positive alteration in the individual's behaviour as well as in their attitude towards their diabetes self-management. Assistive technologies such as flash glucose sensor testing is now widely available for everyone with diabetes to help manage the condition more effectively. This, coupled with specific information, education and support from a number of sources, means that managing diabetes well in the 21st century is highly achievable.

Key messages in this chapter:

- Concordance refers to the extent an individual follows a given medical treatment regime. The term 'non-concordance' is used to describe individuals who do not follow the advice of healthcare professionals.
- Concordance is a behaviour that does not remain the same over time: concordance increases with duration of diabetes.
- Although empowerment – informed choice – supports concordance and does not associate non-concordance with following a diabetes self-management regime, the individual may decide not to – or not be able to – fully concur with medical advice.
- The Diabetes Control and Complications Trial for Type 1 diabetes, and the UK Prospective Diabetes Study for Type 2 diabetes, showed that intensive diabetes self-management using either multiple daily insulin injections or insulin pump therapy is essential in reducing the risk of micro- and macrovascular complications.
- Locus of control describes the individual's perception of a stressful event and its impact on subsequent behaviour: locus of control may be internal or external.
- Motivation – a key element of the COM-B model of behaviour – is defined in psychological terms as internal processes that spur us on to satisfy some need. Perceived vulnerability to complications and a high degree of self-efficacy are the motivational drives for effective diabetes self-care.
- Self-efficacy is defined as a particular set of beliefs that determine how well an individual can carry out a specific positive health behaviour. Self-efficacy and motivation underpin intention to undertake a specific behaviour.

3 Theories of Behaviour Applied to Diabetes

Behaviour is key to the successful self-management of diabetes, although this complex area is often overlooked. Diabetes presents a behavioural challenge to both the individual and their healthcare team, with effective management of the condition being dependent on the initiation and maintenance of a composite series of behaviours. Health behaviours are defined as 'behaviour patterns, actions and habits that relate to health maintenance, to health restoration and to health improvement' (Gochman, 1997). These patterns have a vast ability to positively or negatively impact an individual's health. Much theoretical research has attempted to explain human behaviour in terms of how individuals react when told they have a chronic health condition, and how they go on to manage that condition.

Type 1 diabetes self-management

Type 1 diabetes requires adoption of a comprehensive self-management routine including multiple daily insulin injections, or insulin pump therapy use, regular blood glucose self-monitoring throughout the day and often during the night, and continual observance of diet and exercise. This high degree of continual self-care required – unlike any other chronic health condition – is carried out by the individual themselves to achieve near-normal blood glucose levels between 4.0–7.0 mmol/L (or 72–126 mg/dl US measurement).

In some instances, however, Type 1 diabetes is very difficult to self-manage because good glycaemic control cannot be easily achieved – termed 'brittle' diabetes. An individual may therefore do everything they can to manage their condition to the best of their abilities, but still not achieve this goal. Lack of diabetes control may cause the individual to abandon trying to achieve near-normal blood glucose levels altogether,

DOI: 10.4324/9781003260219-4

or conversely, they may become over-diligent in their attempts to attain better management:

> 'My [Type 1] diabetes has always been really difficult to control, so I inject twice a day and then forget about it: there's nothing I can do that makes any difference'.
>
> 'Although I have very volatile [Type 1] diabetes, I manage it as well as possible with insulin pump therapy and blood testing six times a day. I also use my exercise bike for half an hour in the evening so I don't get a sharp rise in blood glucose after my main meal'.

Type 2 diabetes self-management

Type 2 diabetes is managed with oral anti-hyperglycaemic medication, eating a diet that avoids refined carbohydrates, and by taking moderate, regular exercise. Where oral medication fails to reduce blood glucose levels the individual will also need to take insulin by injection.

Psychosocial and behavioural aspects may differ according to diabetes type. Hempler, et al. (2016) found that individuals with Type 2 diabetes were less physically active and less confident about seeking medical help in the case of serious illness when compared with those with Type 1 diabetes, while males with Type 2 were less likely to follow dietary advice. Following a Type 2 diabetes diagnosis, health behaviours are crucial to patient outcomes. Behaviours such as physical inactivity, poor diet, excessive alcohol consumption and smoking each contribute to the development of diabetes complications. Cardiovascular risk is heightened in Type 2 diabetes, and cardiovascular complications remain the leading cause of morbidity and premature mortality in people with diabetes (Keating, et al., 2016).

Diabetes education approaches

Many of the approaches adopted in diabetes health education research and practice are rooted in the social and behavioural sciences – especially psychology – to determine why some individuals are not positively engaged in their diabetes self-management. Psychological theories are very relevant to diabetes education because they attempt to explain health behaviour and how an individual adapts to any change (Fadhil and

Wang, 2019; Swanson and Maltinsky, 2019; Hood, 2018). As a result, attempts have been made to combine different health behaviour theories – which often have similar concepts, although it has proved difficult to determine the reason why change is made, maintained or may alter. Motivation is influenced by a number of factors including awareness; ability; the individual's social and professional standing; the individual's perceived aptitude; understanding of outcome; objectives; recall; commitment; setting and resources; social motives; emotion; behavioural management, and the type of behaviour.

There is no single theory, framework, or model that can explain the complexities of human behavior. For this reason, it is necessary to combine models in an attempt to improve our understanding of diabetes self-management behaviors – taking medication according to medical advice, regular exercise, healthy diet, etc. – and health outcomes – quality of life, pain, and incapacity. Combined theoretical frameworks may help increase the effectiveness of behavioral interventions by identifying potential treatment targets. Diabetes clinical practice commonly follows two main models of behaviour: the COM-B model of behaviour change and the Common Sense model of illness self-regulation.

Diabetes, the COM-B model and the Behaviour Change Wheel

With the attention on theory, many new behaviour change theories have developed over the past few decades; however, having too many theories has been overwhelming for the design and implementation of behaviour change interventions. The COM-B – Capability, Opportunity, Motivation, Behaviour – model was devised to define the minimum number of features needed to explain behaviour change. In this respect, the COM-B model provides an easy-to-use approach to understanding the context of behaviour over time-honoured theories such as the Stages of Change model (Prochaska and Velicier, 1997). This advantage means that the COM-B model can be quickly assimilated and utilised by healthcare professionals.

Behavioural science has made significant advances in recent years with the development of staged behaviour change guidance, such as the Behaviour Change Wheel (BCW) to summarize theoretical underpinnings including theories of behaviour change, and theoretical constructs including the COM-B model (Michie, et al., 2014) which are used practically in diabetes care. As a systematic approach to intervention design, the Behaviour Change Wheel combines existing behaviour change frameworks. The COM-B model is at the centre of the BCW as the predominant model of behaviour that forms the basis for an intervention.

The COM-B model of behaviour is widely used to identify what needs to change in order for a behaviour modification initiative to be successful, focusing on the individual's capability, opportunity and motivation for that change. Over time, these factors interact so that behaviour can be seen as part of a dynamic structure of positive and negative feedback loops. Motivation is a core principle of the COM-B model and the PRIME Theory of motivation (proposing that every moment is governed by impulses and inhibitions) provides a framework for understanding how reflective thought processes – planning and evaluation – and emotional and habitual processes – motive and impulse/inhibition – interact to trigger behavioural responses at that moment (West and Mitchie, 2020).

The COM-B model comprises three aspects, each with two further components, which interact to influence behaviour:

• capability – physical and psychological
• opportunity – physical and social
• motivation – reflective and automatic

Once a goal behaviour is identified, the COM-B model provides guidance to determine what alteration/s will bring about change. The BCW system then provides the means to match the COM-B components to intervention categories so an intervention can change behaviour, such as education, environmental restructuring and incentives. The COM-B model and BCW has proved successful in identifying barriers to effective Type 1 diabetes self-management in young adults (Stanton-Fey, et al., 2021) and for diabetic individuals under 40 years of age regarding taking up retinal screening appointments (Michie, et al, 2014).

Critique of the COM-B model and Behaviour Change Wheel

While the COM-B and BCW are frequently used, these approaches have been accused of being too simplistic and systematic, suggesting that the COM-B model does not explain all types of behaviour with enough intensity (Ogden, 2016; Peters and Kok, 2016). There is also no evidence that these approaches are more effective than older models used to explain behaviour, such as the Stages of Change model (Prochaska and Velicier, 1997), or the Health Belief model (Becker and Janz, 1985). The

COM-B and BCW therefore provide suggestions to interpret behaviour rather than being replacement theories for the more traditional models.

Empowerment is an important concept in diabetes self-care and yet, the COM-B model – used to identify what needs to change in order for a behaviour modification to be successful – and the BCW – used to match the COM-B components to intervention categories – have been criticised for their reduced emphasis on diabetes empowerment and self-determination. These approaches aim to achieve behaviour change according to what healthcare professionals or the intervention designers suggest is the correct behaviour rather than what the individual can achieve. Michie, et al, (2014) states that these models can be successfully used in both one-to-one and group-centred interventions to support behaviour change, although the individual may be unable or unwilling to alter their behaviour.

Diabetes and the Common Sense model

The Common Sense model of self-regulation emerged from research examining the effect of fear on health behaviors (Leventhal, 1970). The CSM has developed into a widely-used framework for understanding how individuals construct illness representations in response to health threats such as diabetes and its complications. With similar concepts to the Health Belief model (1985), the CSM of illness self-regulation (Leventhal, et al., 1980; Leventhal, et al., 1984) suggests that beliefs about illness have five basic concepts: cause; identity; perceived control; severity of illness consequences, and time line. Subsequent research has added further concepts to this set of illness beliefs, including illness coherence – a belief that the illness 'makes sense' (Moss-Morris, et al., 2002).

Greater emotional distress in diabetes is associated with poorer self-care and impaired metabolic control. Paddison, et al., (2010) examined the relationships between illness perceptions and illness-related distress in adults with Type 2 diabetes. Adults with diabetes are twice as likely to be depressed than similar individuals without diabetes (Anderson, et al., (2001) and depression is strongly associated with poor glycaemic control (Lustman, et al., 2000). The Diabetes Attitudes, Wishes and Needs (DAWN) Study (Peyrot, et al., 2005) found healthcare professionals believed that psychological problems affected their patients' diabetes self-management behaviour. Poor access to, and engagement with, diabetes healthcare is a significant issue for black British communities who are disproportionately diagnosed with Type 2 diabetes. Provision of culturally sensitive diabetes care and behaviour change interventions remains a challenging area of practice for healthcare professionals, who recognise the need for more training and resources to support them in developing cultural competence (Goff, et al., 2020).

In terms of the individual's perceived control of their diabetes, or potential outcomes due to severity of illness, the CSM suggests that illness perceptions ultimately influence emotional outcomes such as illness-related distress. Diabetes-related distress is determined by the number of symptoms perceived as being due to the condition and the individual's ability to adjust to these challenges (Paschalides, et al., 2004; Edgar and Skinner, 2003). This includes the perceived consequences of these health issues, such as depression and anxiety (Law, et al., 2002). The Common Sense model has been successfully used with older adults who have Type 2 diabetes (Grzywacz, et al., 2012) and in young persons with Type 1 diabetes (Huston and Houk, 2011).

Critique of the Common Sense model

The CSM continues to advance, with additions such as recognition of the need for multiple means of assessing illness representations beyond the predominantly verbal assessments currently used (Broadbent, et al., 2019). It is the case that some illness representations cannot be categorised – medically unexplained symptoms – which impact on quality of life by causing distress (McAndrew, et al., 2019). This perceived threat reverts to the original Leventhal (1970) fear of illness principle. Although difficult to measure, it should be recognised that regulation of diabetes self-management behaviour is heavily influenced by automatic processes of illness recognition and identification, with relevant learned responses. With this in mind, it may be inappropriate to initiate unconscious processes as a means to achieving behaviour change (Orbell and Phillips, 2019).

Self-Regulation Theory and Perpetual Control Theory

Two further interventions involving goal-setting and action planning in order to change behaviour are Self-Regulation Theory (SRT) and Perpetual Control Theory (PCT). SRT is a system of conscious personal management that involves the process of guiding one's own thoughts, behaviors and feelings to reach goals, including impulse control and the management of short-term desires – people with low impulse control are prone to acting on immediate desires. PCT is a model of behavior based on the principles of negative feedback.

These theories focus on personally-defined goals rather than a target set by a healthcare professional for the individual to aspire to. Self-Regulation Theory suggests that the individual reflects on their progress, disseminating this information back to the healthcare professionals providing their care because it can help maintain a change in weight or blood pressure, while PCT encourages the individual to identify negative behaviours, similar to the principle of Cognitive Behaviour Therapy. However, this reflection and emphasis on improvement may actually be de-motivating if blood glucose levels are not improved as a result, despite self-care efforts. This is especially the case when blood glucose levels are increased due to stress or depression and the biological and psychological factors affecting glucose metabolism. Depression interacts negatively with diabetes, leading to erratic diabetes control and a 1.8 per cent increase in HbA1c.

Conclusion

Altering unhealthy behaviours – such as non-engagement in regular blood glucose monitoring, avoiding exercise, poor dietary choices, smoking and excessive alcohol consumption – is central to improving diabetes care outcomes. Behaviour change is also an important personal consideration for health professionals delivering diabetes care. Despite this recognition, many behaviour change attempts only achieve partial success, due to a lack of time, resources or understanding of behaviour change.

Behavioural science approaches have been modified since Leventhal first proposed his model of illness self-regulation (1970) to reflect a greater number of concepts in the understanding of illness perception and behaviour. The challenge for the future is to increase the adoption of these theoretical approaches in the delivery of diabetes care with professional guidelines to ensure maximum impact on the health and wellbeing of people with diabetes.

Key messages in this chapter

- Individuals with diabetes provide 95 percent (or more) of their own care.
- The Department of Health National Service Framework for Diabetes states that diabetes self-management is the key to good diabetes care. The document suggests that this can be achieved by the individual with the provision of information, education and psychological support from healthcare professionals.

- There is no single theory, framework, or model that can explain the complexities of human behavior.
- The COM-B – Capability, Opportunity, Motivation, Behaviour – model was devised to define the minimum number of features needed to explain behaviour change, providing an easy-to-use approach to understanding the context of behaviour.
- The Behaviour Change Wheel system provides the means to match the COM-B components to intervention categories so an intervention can change behaviour, such as education, environmental restructuring and incentives.
- The Common Sense model is a widely-used framework for understanding how individuals construct illness representations in response to health threats such as diabetes and its complications.

4　Diabetes and Depression

Psychological disorders can be especially devastating for individuals with diabetes; as we have already seen, episodes of depression appear to be more frequent and severe than in the general population. In addition, all of the most common mental health disorders – such as depression, anxiety, phobias, seasonal affective disorder, eating disorders and obsessive-compulsive disorder – can interfere with diabetes management. Reductions in self-care contribute to elevated blood glucose levels, significantly increasing the risk of acute and long-term diabetes complications and leading to a worsened quality of life.

Diabetes associated with mental health conditions

There is an established association between Type 2 diabetes and psychotic disorders, with an increased level of diabetes occurring with first-episode psychosis. Anti-psychosis medication leads to weight gain and decreased insulin sensitivity, increasing the risk of developing Type 2 diabetes (Neuvo, et al., 2011; Baker, et al., 2009).

When there is diabetic ketoacidosis – predominantly in Type 1 diabetes and more rarely in Type 2 – acid by-products are formed that, in large quantities, cause the blood to become acidic. This state of acid-imbalance is known to trigger chronic complications, such as retinopathy (Russell, 2012). Ketoacidosis is the major cause of mortality in people with Type 1 diabetes because the condition leads to circulatory collapse, low serum potassium levels and swelling of the brain, known as cerebral oedema (Katsilambros, et al., 2011). Diabetic ketoacidosis may also be the underlying cause of a heart attack in individuals with Type 2 diabetes.

Aliyu (2015) reported the case of an 11-year-old child with Type 1 diabetes who became unconscious and developed schizophrenia following an episode of severe DKA. Whilst being treated in hospital for

DOI: 10.4324/9781003260219-5

DKA after regaining consciousness, the young patient suddenly developed visual hallucinations, irrational conversation, aggressive behaviour and confused speech and thoughts. The child had no former history of mental health problems, had not sustained head trauma, and had a normal temperature. DKA was reversed and blood and urine tests were normal during the psychotic episode. Anti-psychotic medication – chlorpromazine – resulted in a significant improvement. Aliyu (2015) stated that the child attended follow-up appointments at the hospital and after six months, had experienced no recurrence of the symptoms.

The acute psychosis reported by Aliyu (2015) is associated with metabolic, structural neurologic disorders and diseases such as malaria and typhoid, although it is not known how this occurs (Spelman, et al., 2007; Sowunmi, et al., 1993). It is possible that schizophrenic symptoms presented in the 11-year-old due to a fluid shift in the brain caused by the metabolic imbalance of DKA. Although this is the most likely explanation, glucose, sodium and potassium levels were normal at the time of the psychosis, making it difficult to determine the origin of this episode. However, the association between Type 1 diabetes and psychosis is rare (Aliyu, 2015).

Depression

Depression is a common and very serious medical condition with a lifetime prevalence, although alternating emotions are normal. The association between diabetes and mental health problems is not a new observation: in the 17th century, Thomas Willis, renowned anatomist and diabetes specialist, stated that, 'Diabetes is a consequence of prolonged sorrow' (Willis, 1675). Evidence shows that the risk of developing a mental health problem over a lifetime is 42 percent for individuals with Type 1 diabetes and 36 percent for those with Type 2 (Perrin, et al., 2017). This has significant consequences such as loss of employment, productivity and income. Depression and anxiety have been cited as the second main cause of disability, while diabetes is the eighth major cause of disability – adjusted for life years – in developed countries.

There is a correlation between the burden and severity of comorbid illness, such as depression and diabetes, and suicide (The Mental Health Foundation, 2020; Ikeda, et al., 2001). Depression is also associated with increased medical morbidity – how often a disease occurs, and mortality – the number of deaths from a given cause. Carney and Freedland (2003) found that individuals with depression who had suffered a myocardial infarction – damaging a portion of the heart due to poor or absent blood supply – were significantly more likely to have future coronary events and death compared to individuals without depression.

There is a 2 percent higher risk of death from all causes for individuals with depression compared to those without the condition. Untreated depression brings with it extensive adverse effects – whether this is because the condition has not been diagnosed, or due to non-concordance with a treatment regime, such as anti-depressant medication – with an emphasis on the individual's decreased capacity and functioning, and the heightened risk of suicide and death from all causes.

Depression associated with poor glycaemic control is the most common condition affecting adults and children with diabetes. It is also the case that poorly-managed blood glucose levels and prolonged hyperglycaemia result in major diabetic complications; greater healthcare costs; increased functional disability; frequent hospitalisation, and premature mortality (Holt, et al., 2014). However, as we have already seen, depression is not purely related to the burden of having diabetes and its necessary self-care requirements.

Those individuals with psychological distress at the time their diabetes is diagnosed are one-and-a-half times more likely to experience cardiovascular complications, and are twice as likely to die than diabetes patients without psychological illness (Dalsgaard, et al., 2014). This highlights the adverse effects of physical and psychological changes that occur before diabetes is diagnosed. As previously mentioned, Diabetes UK (2008) found that Type 2 diabetes may remain undiagnosed for up to 12 years because the symptoms are mild, but elevated blood glucose levels over this period damage minor and major blood vessels, meaning that unrecognised Type 2 diabetes presents a significant risk to vascular health.

Major depression is thought to be the second leading cause of disability worldwide and mental health problems are the overall cause of disease burden worldwide (The Metal Health Foundation, 2020). Diabetes and depression occur together approximately twice as frequently as would be expected by chance alone; having diabetes therefore doubles the chance of also developing depression. According to the International Diabetes Federation, diabetes is one of the greatest global health emergencies of the 21st century (International Diabetes Federation, 2015). When this statement was made in 2015, the prevalence of diabetes worldwide was one in every 11 adults and the estimated prevalence of poor diabetes management among those with the condition was one in 15 adults. These figures are continually escalating – especially with the huge global rise in Type 2 diabetes – increasing medical and economic burden. If the number of individuals worldwide with pre-diabetes – not yet full-blown Type 2 – is added, this creates a significant clinical issue, where psychological needs can never be fully met.

Effects of depression on diabetes self-care

Without doubt, the presence of depression adversely affects diabetes both physiologically and psychologically. The burden of depression negatively affects the reporting of any symptoms associated with diabetes to healthcare professionals; it reduces the individual's concordance with medical advice and diabetes self-care behaviour, leading to poor gly-caemic control over an extended period (De Groot, et al., 2001). High blood glucose levels over time significantly increase the risk of devel-oping chronic complications of diabetes, such as blindness, limb am-putation and kidney failure. The myriad effects of depression on diabetes should not be under-estimated by either the individual or by healthcare professionals.

It is thought that one in four individuals with diabetes have episodes of depression throughout their lifetime. Clark (2004a, 2004b) suggests that diabetes-related depression results from psychological, physical and genetic factors. A number of physical and psychological changes occur in diabetes, causing neurochemical and neurovascular abnormalities that trigger depression; genetic factors also have a role, despite the fact that they may be unrelated to diabetes (Chiba, et al., 2000; Lustman, et al., 1997a; 1992). The extent that these factors contribute to depression in those with diabetes is subjective but the necessity of adopting lifestyle changes, adjustments for dietary restriction and treatment regime, and coping with the ongoing necessity of diabetes self-care takes its toll. Physical impairment due to chronic complications of diabetes such as sight loss due to diabetic retinopathy, or chronic nerve pain due to diabetic neuropathy, also impacts heavily on mental health status.

Not everyone with diabetes will experience a mental health problem, and support needs may change throughout life. For individuals with diabetes in primary care, 4–15 percent meet the criteria for major de-pression and another 9–16 percent meet the criteria for a diagnosis of other psychological disorders, such as anxiety (Diabetes UK, 2016). Clark (2004b) has stated that one-third of individuals with diabetes experience an episode of major depression in their lifetime, a figure higher than for the general population. Older people and individuals with a poor economic status experience particularly high rates of de-pression; these groups are at the highest risk for developing diabetes and its complications (Piette, et al., 2004; De Groot, et al., 2001).

Depression is three times more prevalent in individuals with diabetes when compared with the general population, affecting at least 15 percent of the diabetes population (Clark, 2004a; Peyrot, et al, 1997), although this could be much higher as depression often goes unreported or unrecognised. When compared to rates of mental health disorders among individuals with other chronic illnesses such as arthritis, depression is more prevalent among those with diabetes (Pouwer, et al., 2003). It is also the case that after an initial episode of depression, relapse occurs more frequently for individuals with diabetes than for any other chronic health condition (Clark, 2004b).

As previously mentioned, depression in diabetes leads to poor glycaemic control because of metabolic changes and the individual's inability to carry out certain diabetes self-care activities. Behavioural characteristics manifest, such as negative thought processes; internalising – an internal rather than an external locus of control; pessimistic attributional styles – consistently blaming oneself for negative events, and displaying passive – emotionally-focused – rather than proactive coping strategies (Goodman and Whitaker, 2002; Abramson, et al., 2001).

Negative thought patterns also cause depressed individuals to anticipate that negative events will repeat themselves with the same adverse results; experience of negative events may be carried over into diabetes self-care with a perspective of inability to manage the condition due to depression and situations beyond the individual's control. This mind-set also means that the individual is highly unlikely to follow through any plans for health-related behaviour change as they believe it is unachievable or will be of little value.

Ciechanowski, et al. (2003) and DiMatteo, et al. (2000) identified a causal link between depression and decreased ability in those with chronic illness to carry out their self-care routine. Similarly, McKellar, et al., (2004) reported that a group of individuals with Type 2 diabetes and depression were 50 percent less likely to take their diabetes medication compared with those with no depressive symptoms. Conversely, individuals who have experienced remission of their depression are known to experience a heightened sense of self-efficacy, enabling them to undertake more diabetes self-care activities which is associated with improved glycaemic control.

The physical and healthcare costs of depression

Major depression has a huge impact on all aspects of the individual's health and social situation. This includes functional disability and absence from work, higher education or school, as well as increased healthcare expenditure. Holt, et al. (2014) suggest that depression in those with diabetes is recurrent and more severe when compared with the general population and that less than 10 percent of individuals will remain symptom free for longer than 5 years. It is thought that depression occurs more often in women than in men with diabetes – which is equally true in the general population, with rates of depression being similar for Type 1 and Type 2 diabetes (Anderson, et al., 2001; Talbot and Nouwen, 2000). In the UK, NHS service usage for individuals with diabetes increased from an average of £3,910 per annum, per person to £5,670 when the cost of treating mental health problems is included (Naylor, et al., 2012).

As we have seen, due to the metabolic imbalance that diabetes imposes, normal brain function is impeded by hypo– or hyperglycaemia which disrupts the fine balance of glucose used for fuel; too much glucose in the blood is toxic to the brain. It is reasonable to assume that this imbalance triggers chemical changes in the brain and depressive symptoms. In 2014, the Endocrine Society confirmed a biological link between hyperglycaemia and depression in people with Type 1 diabetes, where as little as a 1.8 percent increase in HbA1c glycosylated haemoglobin has been shown to cause depressive symptoms.

The UK Prospective Diabetes Study (1998a; 1998b) found that 49 percent of those with Type 2 diabetes taking insulin and 56 percent of those taking diabetes medication had HbA1c values of 8.0 percent or higher – 6.0 to 6.5 percent being the recommendation in the UK and an average of <7.0 percent in the United States. Depression can therefore be regarded as both a condition in its own right and a complication of diabetes; it is triggered or worsened by poor glycaemic control in the same way as physical complications such as retinopathy, neuropathy, nephropathy and circulatory system complications.

In a feedback loop, depression has been directly linked to the development of neuropathy and cardiovascular disease (Clark, 2004a), having direct and indirect links to glycaemic control and diabetes complications in adults and adolescents (De Groot, et al., 2001; Lustman, et al., 2000a). The link between depression, glycaemic control and complications can be seen in the following comment:

> 'When I'm depressed the neuropathy in my feet and legs is worse, even if my blood glucose levels are OK. It's usually worse at night, with sharp pains in my calves and periodic prickling and numbness in the soles of my feet and toes. I don't get continuous pain, but if it happens five or six times in the night with sharp little jabs, this keeps me awake, so I feel even worse'.

Depression is also a risk factor for developing hypertension (Davidson, et al., 2000); high levels of harmful blood fats – hyperlipidaemia (Gary, et al., 2000), and heart disease (Abramson, et al, 2001). For individuals with diabetes, each of these conditions increases the likelihood of cardiovascular events. The reason these health conditions contribute towards heart disease differs between Type 1 and Type 2 diabetes (Ciechanowski, et al., 2003; Vaccarino, et al., 2001; Jonas, et al., 2000) although this is most likely due to hyperglycaemia.

The individual may live with symptoms of Type 2 diabetes – tiredness, increased thirst, frequent urination, blurred vision, slow healing of wounds, numbness in the feet and legs, and obesity – for many years before consulting a GP. As we have seen, the symptoms of Type 2 diabetes are milder than those of Type 1, meaning Type 2 diabetes may remain undiagnosed for up to 12 years (Diabetes UK, 2008), prolonging hyperglycaemia and significantly contributing towards the prevalence of heart disease and depression in this group. Additionally, higher rates of retinopathy and macrovascular complications such as stroke are present in individuals with diabetes and depression (De Groot, et al., 2001; Cohen, et al., 1997) and depressed individuals report more diabetes-related symptoms (Ciechanowski, et al., 2003).

A sedentary lifestyle and obesity – the two main risk factors for the development of Type 2 diabetes – are also associated with depression, as well as non-concordance with a diabetes treatment regime and medical advice; these lifestyle factors and consequences also impact negatively on glycaemic control. For these reasons, behaviour change interventions are unsuccessful (DiMatteo, et al., 2000) as lifestyle change requires motivation and self-efficacy, driven by the individual's desire to improve health status. Depression undoubtedly opposes personal efforts to achieve good glycaemic control, being clinically relevant in one in three people with diabetes.

Behavioural and physiological interventions to address depression in those with diabetes are ineffective and equally unsatisfactory. The

Diabetes UK (2016) document, 'Diabetes and mental health' reports dangerous and fatal instances of 'diagnostic over-shadowing' where a mental health treatment did not recognise the risk or presence of diabetes emergencies such as severe low blood glucose levels or diabetic ketoacidosis. Because of the difficulties in matching a suitable depression treatment approach to the individual's needs, medical conditions and current prescribed medications, the condition often goes undiagnosed, and two out of every three cases of depression in those with diabetes are left untreated by primary care physicians (Clark, 2004b). Diabetes-related distress and depression are two separate mental health conditions requiring different treatments.

'I've had Type 1 diabetes for over thirty years and I've suffered all my life from depression. My GP started me on anti-depressants, but they made me feel spaced out like a zombie and I couldn't distinguish this from hypoglycaemia symptoms. I was told that if I wanted Cognitive Behavioural Therapy or counselling, I'd have to pay for it privately because this was not available through the NHS'.

'It took years to get a referral to a clinical psychologist after an NHS psychiatrist said that (as I was dressed in a brightly-coloured skirt and blouse) I couldn't possibly have depression. After seeing the psychologist weekly for a year during which suicide attempts were discussed, I was told that by having an insulin pump attached to me 24/7, I had the ideal portable method to easily kill myself. He also said that if I did want to commit suicide, I should go ahead and try it as it would make me question my motives for doing so'.

Quality of life

Quality of life is directly affected by depression for individuals coping with chronic illness, including diabetes. Because depression negatively affects mental health, it compromises every aspect of life more than physical health conditions such as high blood pressure, chronic lung diseases, gastrointestinal disorders and arthritis (Druss, et al., 2000). Although studies by Lustman (2000b; 1997c) have shown that glycaemic control is only slightly improved by the treatment of depression and can potentially be worsened by it, the individual's quality of life is undoubtedly improved by the remission of depressive symptoms.

There is a correlation between depression in those with diabetes and an increase in reported functional limitations (Ciechanowski, et al., 2003; 2000). In such cases, an increase in physical activity may be an effective form of behavioral change for individuals with diabetes and depression; other studies show a link between physical inactivity, poor quality of life; depression and diabetes (Piette, et al., 2004; Biddle, et al., 2000; Hassmen, et al., 2000). Individuals engaging in regular physical activity are able to achieve better metabolic control and therefore experience fewer depressive symptoms or a faster recovery from an episode of major depression. Undertaking exercise, however, is reliant on the individual's knowledge that reduced physical activity majorly increases the risk of depression (Biddle, et al., 2000).

Interventions to treat depression alone are ineffective, although exercise programmes for people with diabetes and depression are beneficial and improve quality of life. Boule, et al., (2001) found that participants in these exercise programmes had an average HbA1c level of 7.7 percent compared with 8.3 percent for a comparison group who did not exercise. The benefits of taking regular moderate exercise reduced cardiovascular risk factors such as high-density lipoprotein, cholesterol and blood pressure levels. Sirey, et al., (2001b) examined depression in elderly individuals with diabetes. The researchers found that regular exercise resulted in the participants being 50 percent less likely to have depression after 5 months of increased physical activity compared with participants in a similar group who did not exercise. These studies suggest that exercise is a vital component in treating and managing depression and improving quality of life, especially where the suspected cause is hyperglycaemia.

The communication process

Communicating well can change behaviour, even for the most unappealing subject. Satisfaction with patient/provider communication is a strong predictor of concordance with a diabetes medical regime and good metabolic control. Wilson (2003a) found that satisfaction with diabetes care involves a number of factors, such as good patient/provider communication, the ability to speak to a diabetes consultant or nurse when necessary, and the availability of a counsellor/clinical psychologist as part of the diabetes team to address mental health needs.

'When I see my consultant, depression stops me thinking straight; remembering what I want to say, being able to discuss something, or even just answering questions about my diabetes. I then get angry with myself, especially when I've forced myself to go to the appointment. There have been a couple of times when I've thought, "What's the point? I'll just be told I haven't looked after my diabetes very well." That makes me annoyed that they don't recognising my difficulties and help me'.

If an individual perceives that their own agenda is often overlooked they are, understandably, less satisfied with their diabetes care. This is also the case in general medicine, where individuals with this perception are less likely to follow a treatment regime or medical advice and have poorer outcomes. A further study of those with diabetes showed that both good general communication and diabetes-specific communication from health professionals is needed (Piette, et al., 2003). This was also found to be the case by Wilson (2003a) in a study of perceived needs of individuals with Type 1 diabetes.

'I hate being quizzed about my diabetes and how I look after myself. I just do my injections then forget about it. I saw my consultant not long ago and told him I try not to let my diabetes control my life. I got a look of disapproval and was told that my HbA1c was twice what it should be'.

Diabetes requires visits to a number of healthcare professionals, for example, the ophthalmologist for eye checks and the chiropodist/podiatrist for foot care, as well as the diabetes care team, GP and GP Practice nurse. For those with multiple chronic health conditions, their medical history must be recited multiple times, allowing a potential breakdown in communication: this is often perceived by the individual as tiresome, and by healthcare professionals as disinterest (Wilson, 2003a). This could be explained by the individual's high expectation of a non-diabetes healthcare professional's knowledge, followed by disappointment when that professional does not demonstrate understanding from a diabetes perspective.

'The only reason I attend appointments is because I think I'll get the help I need. They don't understand how depression affects me and they haven't got the right attitude or the right thing to say. Usually, I end up feeling very upset afterwards because someone has said something insensitive or uncaring like, "You could do a lot more to help yourself by looking after your diabetes". I've never been offered any practical advice or coping strategies, I'm just left to struggle on my own to try and manage. This makes me very angry as they just don't get it'.

'I went to a hospital eye check appointment for retinopathy and the consultant asked me how my diabetes was. I told her I had a lot of difficulty managing my diabetes and depression. That was the extent of the conversation. I then received a copy of her 'findings' at the appointment and she said she'd advised me on the importance of good blood glucose and cholesterol control, which simply wasn't true'.

Depression may lead to further patient/provider dissatisfaction because of negative thought processes or because of poorer communication. Katon (2003) suggests that individuals with depression are more likely to have unmet expectations after engaging in communication with healthcare professionals, whilst Haviland, et al. (2001) stated that depressed patients are generally less satisfied with the overall medical care they receive.

From the healthcare professional's perspective, individuals with complex needs may be beyond their remit if they are not trained in psychological approaches. Jackson and Kroenke (1999) found that primary care providers are more likely to consider individuals with depressive or anxiety disorders to be 'difficult' and consequently, consider those who have diabetes and depression or anxiety as less able to cope with their diabetes. Similarly, thirty years ago, Petty, et al. (1991) examined the communication process between diabetes consultants and their patients, finding that depression and/or anxiety was perceived as a major limiting factor in effectively self-managing diabetes. This perception ultimately influenced the communication process and also the consultant's management style. Such attitudes may be evidence-based according to HbA1c levels and observed poor self-care. There is also a correlation between individuals with a 'dismissive' interpersonal communication style with healthcare professionals and poor metabolic control (Piette, et al., 2003; Ciechanowski, et al., 2001).

Research has shown that individuals with depression use more healthcare resources and therefore cost more than non-depressed patients (Diabetes UK, 2016). This is perhaps an obvious conclusion when considering that individuals without healthcare needs may rarely visit their GP, let alone a hospital consultant. The subsequent increased healthcare costs of depression and diabetes may be due to poor self-care, low concordance with treatment advice, and difficult interactions with healthcare professionals. In the United States, Ciechanowski, et al. (2000) showed that diabetes and depression had healthcare costs that were 86 percent higher than those of non-depressed individuals with diabetes. Similarly, Egede, et al. (2002) found that healthcare costs for diabetes and depression were 4.5 times higher than those for non-depressed individuals, and that the groups differed in treatment costs even after adjusting for demographic characteristics, health insurance, and coexisting illnesses.

Good communication involves the healthcare professional's innate persuasiveness, the type of message that needs to be imparted and the characteristics of the message recipient. A health education message needs to be believable and the message-giver needs to know the subject matter well. For the patient, a well-directed question about their diabetes self-management is more impressive and persuasive than an observation about the number of diabetic complications the individual has; patients do not tend to react well to being talked down to or a healthcare professional they've never met pointing out what's what. A health education message must be delivered confidently but not over-confidently and if the message is complex, the first and last points made tend to be the ones that are remembered. Therefore, stating the main message points in more than one way in addition to giving a summary allows the patient to remember what they have been told. Communicating a message that is not too far from pre-held health beliefs will effectively encourage the patient in the desired direction.

Identifying depression in individuals with diabetes

The diagnosis of major depressive disorder is made when the symptoms occur together, when they are severe, and when they persist daily for a minimum of two weeks (American Psychiatric Association, 2013). Although symptoms may vary, generalised sadness for no specific reason and lack of interest in pleasurable activities are key diagnostic signs. The symptoms must be categorised as distressing to the individual, or must cause a decline in social, occupational or other key functions to constitute a diagnosis of depression; symptoms that result from taking illicit drugs or prescription medication, or that arise from bereavement are not counted (Clark, 2004b). Unfortunately, mental health symptoms due to diabetes – such as the burden of self-care – are also not recognised in making a diagnosis of depression, meaning that the emotional and physical impact of diabetes is discounted.

Although omitting coping with a chronic medical condition as an indicator of diabetes-related depression appears counter-productive, this is in place because the symptoms of poorly-controlled diabetes are very similar to those of depression. Feeling constantly 'down', unhappy, listless, tired, un-motivated, disconnected, withdrawn, and irritable – to name but a few symptoms of both conditions – can often be overlooked by healthcare professionals when the individual also has an elevated HbA1c. Diabetes does not directly cause the key symptoms of depression and this practice avoids the over-diagnosis of depression in the diabetes population, reducing the likelihood of a false-positive diagnosis (Clark, 2004a). However, Clark states that poorly-controlled diabetes should not impair the clinician's ability to diagnose depression. Despite this, diabetes associated depression is recognised and treated in less than a third of individuals (Lustman, et al, 2000a).

In spite of the potential benefit of treatment, individuals with diabetes and depression often experience significant gaps in their depression care. As we have already seen, research shows that healthcare professionals often fail to detect depression among their patients and when the condition is identified, depression-specific treatments are not appropriately initiated. Primary care health professionals treating individuals with diabetes may lack expertise in mental health issues or have insufficient time to fully explore depressive symptoms. It is also the case that Cognitive Behavioural Therapy – CBT – is unavailable in certain areas of the country because of the lack of adequately trained therapists, or it is not prescribed due to perceived limitations on mental health benefits (van Bastelaar, et al., 2008).

Barriers to recovery

Long-term concordance with medical advice for individuals taking medication to treat depression is often poor. Van Servellen, et al. (2011) reported that in a large care organisation, 28 percent of patients discontinued their anti-depressant medication within the first month of treatment, with 44 percent discontinuing treatment by the third month. In the United States, medical insurance claim data suggests that up to 70 percent of individuals failed to collect their monthly prescription in the 6 months following initiation of anti-depressant treatment (Shan Xing, et al., 2011).

> 'My depression has badly affected me and some days, I struggle to get out of bed and do the simplest chores. I was referred for CBT by my GP, who thought it would help me manage my diabetes, but I felt ashamed to actually attend. I felt like everyone at the surgery knew why I was going to the hospital and I didn't want to tell anyone I knew in case they judged me. If I said I was going to the diabetes clinic, it wouldn't have been an issue, but a mental health problem made a big difference – my family, friends and work colleagues don't understand as they've never been depressed'.

Individuals with diabetes and depression may feel a certain stigma about 'being observed' in a mental health setting, making them less likely to engage in discussion about treatment for their condition. Sirey, et al. (2001a) suggest that psychological barriers to treatment, such as perceived stigma and the individual's minimisation of their care needs can be significant obstacles to taking medication for major depression. Individuals who have mental ill-health have reported being shunned and avoided by work colleagues and friends (Sakyi, et al., 2015).

> 'I've had a lot of problems coping with depression. My GP suggested I should tell people what I'm going through as they would understand and support me; he was wrong. I told a friend I'd known for many years and she had even worked for a mental health charity at one time, so I thought she'd be a good person to tell – but it was as though we were suddenly strangers. She dropped me like a hot potato, refusing to have any more contact with me. It was like she thought I was disgusting and weak for having depression, as though I'd done something terrible, rather than it being something I have no control over'.
>
> 'I find that people seem to understand when you tell them you have depression, but expect it to be gone quickly – like a cold. When it re-occurs or is worse, they sort of roll their eyes in a, "Here we go again" way'.

Individuals may also be unwilling to undertake a course of treatment for depression because of concerns about stigma or any sideeffects. Treatment to bring depression under control is effective in the short-term if properly followed; however, treatment may be stopped at this point because the clinician or the individual believes depression is no longer present. Additionally, the individual may not wish to undertake the treatment, either because they perceive the regime to be complex, due to medication side-effects, or for other reasons such as stigma and how others perceive them. Unfortunately, research has shown that as few as 40 percent of individuals with diabetes remain free of major depressive disorder in the year following successful initial treatment, with recurrence of symptoms frequently accompanied by a deterioration in glycemic control (Williams, et al., 2006).

Psychosocial circumstances are personal to the individual and a sta-bilised mental health status may deteriorate due to factors such as re-lationship breakdown or bereavement. Research by Weiden, et al. (1997) explains some of these aspects in the context of having a mental health condition and following treatment guidelines, stating that per-ceived stigma from others and the individual's denial of their illness were associated majorly with non-concordance in a group of persons with schizophrenia. It has also been shown that older adults diagnosed with depression often felt highly stigmatised by their illness (Sirey, et al., 2001b), perceiving that they should be able to cope and 'pull themselves together', making them more likely to discontinue their depression treatment.

Individuals with a lower perception of stigma and a higher self-rated severity of illness are more concordant with depression treatment than those who feel highly stigmatised and who report a lower severity of illness. Sirey, et al. (2001b) found that emphasising the need for anti-depressant treatment with older individuals significantly enhanced con-cordance with the treatment regime. Those over 60 years of age were found to be more concordant than younger individuals; while those with personality disorders – such as schizophrenia – were less likely to follow medical advice about their treatment. Severity of depression, functional limitations, or the number of visits to healthcare professionals also did not predict concordance. The expectation of treatment side-effects or any distress caused by side-effects was not found to predict concordance with medical advice. Similar findings have been seen in studies ex-amining diabetes regime concordance, where older individuals and those with chronic complications were more concordant than the newly-diagnosed (Donnovan, et al., 2002).

Self-reporting of concordance with both a diabetes regime and with taking anti-depressant medication is often shown to be good when based on pill counts; however, self-reports may be unreliable as deception, misunderstanding of the regimen, and poor recall must be accounted for. As previously discussed, health beliefs about following a medical regime – and taking anti-depressant medication correctly – is an important factor in predicting health-related behaviors. The Health Belief model has been used to describe health behaviours such as the use of preventive health measures and concordance with a medical regime once ill-health is diagnosed in order to restore health or prevent further illness, rather than for chronic health conditions. This model suggests that perception of the severity of an illness is a major influence on subsequent health behaviour. However, the individual may be in denial when they are told they have depression, and this denial may ultimately override the severity of the illness.

A further potential barrier to effective depression management is the lack of a unifying view of clinical problems that encompass both diabetes and depression; this may involve a lack of collaboration between diabetes care and mental health services. It may also be the case that the diabetes team is located in the hospital setting whilst mental health services are community-based, not operating in the same setting. This situation causes communication difficulties, such as having two sets of patient records and the need for the individual to repeat information to different teams of healthcare professionals. Piette, et al. (2004) stated that primary care providers often do not appreciate the importance of aggressive depression management for overall health, and that individuals often fail to make connections between their depressive symptoms and ability to manage their diabetes. Although the presentation of depression in those with diabetes is well-documented, as is the availability of suitable treatments, there is little consensus regarding how these co-existing conditions should be effectively managed.

In addition to the desire not to over-diagnose depression in diabetes that leads to the condition frequently going unrecognised, it is important to distinguish depression as a condition in its own right. Because depression interacts very negatively with diabetes there is a tendency to treat only the medical illness rather than the medical and mental health condition. The Beck Depression Inventory (BDI) has been used as a preliminary method in the outpatient setting to identify individuals with depressive symptoms. This 21-question patient-completed survey involves summing ratings for each question. A score of >16 identifies a major depressive disorder and this inventory has been very successful in determining depression in over 70 percent of patients (Garcia-Batista, et al., 2019). It has also been suggested that two particular areas of questioning – for example, 'How have you been feeling recently? Have you been low in spirits?', and, 'Have you been able to enjoy the things you usually enjoy?' – can determine major depression in up to 95 percent of individuals (Peveler, et al., 2002).

As well as the Beck Depression Inventory, the Center for Epidemiologic Studies Depression Scale is used to identify depression. When using both the Beck Depression Inventory and the Center for Epidemiologic Studies in Depression Scale in different research studies, depression prevalence was found to be equal to the number of subjects with scores above a specified value.

Treatment and management

In the short-term, the individual presenting with both diabetes and major depression requires specific therapeutic intervention as little improvement is seen with non-specific measures (Williams, et al., 2006). Both psychotherapy and anti-depressant medication are effective treatments for depression in this situation (Clark, 2004b; Lustman, et al., 2000a). Medication has the advantage over psychotherapy in primary care because it does not require the time and expertise of a healthcare professional to administer, costing the healthcare provider less. Some anti-depressant medications, however, have undesirable side-effects which exacerbate the difficulties of managing diabetes effectively.

> 'I've tried various anti-depressant tablets and they all make me feel really groggy. The trouble is, I can't detect symptoms of hypoglycaemia if I take these pills because feeling disorientated and confused with a bad headache and a muzzy head – how the medication makes me feel – are exactly the same symptoms as hypoglycaemia'.

Management guidelines only provide a framework for treating diabetes as the primary condition and not coexisting conditions such as depression. Depression comes under the broad area of tailoring the guidelines to the individual's specific needs. This often fails to integrate all care needs – treating mental health issues as only part of the individual rather than how it affects the whole patient in conjunction with other health issues.

Anti-depressant medication

Research examining the treatment of depression in diabetes with medication has reported absolute increases in remission rates of 17–39 percent (Piette, et al., 2004). This is confirmed when comparing individuals receiving anti-depressants with those receiving a placebo (Snow, et al., 2000). Anti-depressant medication is as effective for individuals with comorbid medical conditions as for those with major depression alone (Gill and Hatcher, 2000). The type of medication depends on the range of presenting symptoms, other medical conditions, potential contraindications – drug interactions between existing medication(s) – and any side-effects.

Tricyclic anti-depressants are a range of medications – such as Nortriptyline, having the added advantage of regulating sleep. An unfortunate side-effect of some anti-depressant medications for those with diabetes is weight gain and adverse cardiovascular effects (Clark, 2004b). Other depression medications are selective serotonin re-uptake inhibitors, such as Fluoxetine, which Lustman, et al. (2000b) suggest is particularly effective in the treatment of depression for people with diabetes. SSRIs have the added advantage that they do not lead to weight gain or sedation; however, they do have side-effects such as gastrointestinal upset, agitation and sexual dysfunction.

Gastrointestinal disturbance may be mistaken for diabetic diarrhoea – due to autonomic neuropathy, and sexual dysfunction can be attributed to diabetes-related impotence. The Type 2 diabetes medication, Metformin causes diarrhoea in 10 percent of individuals, with incontinence being one of the commonest side-effects.

Because there is no need for a trained therapist and the lower cost of anti-depressant medication in primary care, SSRIs such as Bupropion, Mirtazapine and Venlafaxine are used as an initial treatment for individuals with depression and diabetes (Williams, et al., 2006; Lustman, et al., 2006; 1997a). Bupropion is less likely to cause weight gain or sexual dysfunction and does not cause gastrointestinal disturbance. These benefits over other anti-depressant medications may encourage greater tolerance of an anti-depressant medication regime (Lustman, et al., 2002). The following comment gives an example of why anti-depressant medication is prescribed but not taken by the individual.

'I was prescribed Amitriptyline as I have severe back pain; the consultant told me it would also help my depression. When I read the information leaflet for the tablets, I found that they could increase feelings of suicide, as well as causing major fluctuations in blood glucose levels. I didn't even bother to take one tablet as I'm already depressed enough and have problems with erratic glucose levels'.

The effective management of depression in those with diabetes requires an understanding of both conditions, and any potential contraindications or adverse reactions to medications taken in conjunction with a new treatment. Older treatments for depression, such as monoamine oxidase inhibitors – MOIs – and tricyclic anti-depressants – TCAs – are more dangerous if prescribed dose is exceeded; these have more unpleasant side-effects – such as weight gain and sedation – than newer medications. TCAs have also been associated with orthostatic hypotension – low blood pressure, urinary retention and heart rhythm defects, making them unsuitable for people with cardiovascular disease and diabetes. Before any anti-depressant medication is prescribed a check of current prescriptive medications known to contribute to depression is made. These include some anti-hypertensive drugs to treat high blood pressure; anti-neoplastic medication – preventing abnormal growth of tissue, and immunosuppressant agents prescribed after organ transplant (Brown, et al., 2003).

Psychotherapy

'I've told my GP and diabetes consultant numerus times that I have depression and that's why my blood glucose levels are high; I know that it's depression because I've had it all my life. Sometimes I have weeks that are worse than others, but I get the impression that I'm not being listened to and the GP and diabetes team don't talk to one another. They think I'm just using my depression as an excuse for not looking after my diabetes properly. I always get a lecture on why reducing my glucose levels is important. I know why my diabetes isn't well-controlled, I just can't do it'.

'When I moved to a different area I explained to my new diabetes consultant that I have depression. He looked at me as though I was lying, flicked through my clinic notes and told me I should try harder to look after my diabetes. I was told to go to my new GP for some better [anti-depressive] treatment. The GP hadn't even told him I'd got depression. It feels like neither of them recognise my problem and how it affects my diabetes. Surely I can't be the first person they've ever seen that has diabetes and depression at the same time?'

Approaches such as cognitive behavioural therapy – CBT – or associated therapies such as problem-solving therapy for individuals with depression are effective and beneficial (American Psychiatric Association, 1993). CBT involves a therapist and the individual working together to undo repeated patterns of negative thoughts, low mood, decreased motivation, and inactivity with the aim of increasing pleasurable and productive activities to improve the individual's quality of life. This method of treating depression involves the use of proven techniques that aim to remove depressive symptoms.

The advantage of psychotherapy is that it has no side-effects when used for individuals with diabetes compared with anti-depressant medication. CBT has been shown to be an effective intervention for concordance, depression and glycaemic control, especially in Type 2 diabetes (Safren, et al, 2014). When comparing the effects of CBT and self-management training, Furnes, et al (2014) found that after 10 weeks, remission of depression was 85 percent in patients with Type 2 diabetes treated with a combination of CBT and self-management training, whilst it was only 27 percent in the self-management training group alone. A six-month follow-up found that these rates were 70 percent versus 33.3 percent for the non-CBT group; HbA1c was 9.5 percent for the CBT group and 10.9 percent for the control group who received no psychotherapy treatment. This highlights the adverse relationship between diabetes and depression, where hyperglycaemia remained high during and after CBT, although HbA1c levels were lower than in the control group.

Electro-convulsive therapy – ECT – is only considered for those with severe or life-threatening depression; it is performed on an outpatient basis and provides marked relief from symptoms (Mayo Clinic, 2018). ECT is known to be safe and effective for people with and without diabetes, having no adverse effects on glycaemic control (Netzel, et al.,

2002). This suitability provides an alternative treatment option for those with diabetes and severe depression who suffer side-effects from anti-depressant medications, or for those where medications are contra-indicated. However, a strong anti-ECT lobby is of the opinion that human beings should not be subjected to repeated electric shock to the brain, resulting in distinct adverse after-effects on the personality and cognitive ability.

Treating depression to improve diabetes control

When there is prolonged hyperglycaemia, the amount of blood glucose is raised above normal – recommended levels being 6.0–6.5 percent in the UK and at or <7.0 percent in the United States. Hyperglycaemia and insulin resistance – the need for more insulin to maintain normogly-caemia – are determinants of the onset and progression of diabetes complications (Shaw and Cummings, 2005; De Groot, et al., 2001; DCCT, 1993; UKPDS, 1998a; 1998b). As we have already seen, these targets are rarely met, despite available treatments and good hospital diabetes care.

The effect of depression medication on glucose levels and insulin resistance has been examined. Lustman, et al. (1997c) gave Nortriptyline – an anti-depressant and mild sedative – to depressed and non-depressed individuals to assess any change in HbA1c levels. The medication was shown to worsen glycaemic control, although depressive symptoms were reduced. In a second study, Lustman, et al. (2000b) administered Fluoxetine – an anti-depressant medication with fewer sedative effects – to individuals with and without diabetes, finding that those with diabetes had a reduction in HbA1c levels after 8 weeks of treatment. A third study by Lustman, et al. (2006) showed that Bupropion reduced symptoms of depression in more than 80 percent of patients with Type 2 diabetes; weight loss and depression improvement were also shown to reduce HbA1c levels.

'My GP said I was at high risk of developing Type 2 diabetes as I was overweight, had depression, and a family history of diabetes. A glucose tolerance test showed I was insulin resistant, with high cholesterol and blood pressure levels. This was like a wake-up call as my Mum was almost blind with diabetes and my Dad had a leg amputated because of it. I lost a lot of weight and my depression disappeared. I've just had more blood tests and my glucose and cholesterol are normal, and my blood pressure'.

It has been suggested that a recovery from depression is beneficial to all health-related behaviours, such as partaking in exercise, undertaking appropriate self-care behaviours for chronic conditions such as diabetes, and relating to the physiology of glucose metabolism (Williams, et al., 2006; Musselman, et al., 2003). Depression treatments that do not affect the individual's weight, physical activity, glycaemic control and concordance with a medical regime are paramount. Exercise is a preventative measure in delaying the transition from pre-diabetes to Type 2 diabetes, having the effect of increasing insulin sensitivity. Wiley and Singh (2003) have also suggested that exercise may be particularly useful in helping to prevent recurrent depression in elderly individuals with diabetes.

The presence and treatment of depression symptoms in those with diabetes has a varying impact on the individual's ability to achieve glucose, lipid, and blood pressure targets set by care professionals. Glycaemic targets improve when depression is well-managed with anti-depressants (Lustman, et al., 2006; 2005, 2000a; Clark, 2004b). The achievement of lipid goals – cholesterol and high-density lipids – remains unaffected by the presence of depression symptoms or their treatment (Gary, et al., 2000), although individuals with diabetes and depression are less likely to attend tests for blood fats. Rush, et al. (2008) found that only the systolic rather than the diastolic component of blood pressure testing was better controlled, continuing to improve following a course of anti-depressant treatment.

Treating depression to prevent diabetes

There are inconsistencies concerning whether depression is an independent risk factor for diabetes (Brown, et al., 2005; Carthenon, et al., 2003; Saydah, et al., 2003). The association between diabetes and depression is well-recognised, but the chronology of Type 2 diabetes developing following depression is less well understood (Kessing, et al., 2004; Anderson, et al., 2001). In recent times, however, it has become clear that having a single episode of depression doubles the risk of developing Type 2 diabetes (Williams, et al., 2006; Freedland, 2004), with further evidence suggesting that an episode of depression aged 20–30 years significantly increases the risk of the later development of Type 2 diabetes (Brown, et al., 2005; Weissman, et al., 1996). This knowledge is supported by the evidence that major depressive disorder usually precedes the diagnosis of Type 2 diabetes when the individual is questioned about their medical history (Lustman, et al., 1997). The prevalence of undiagnosed Type 2 diabetes following depression is less easy to define due to the milder nature of diabetes symptoms, meaning that it may not be diagnosed for many years.

Depression is associated with prolonged hyperglycemia in the majority of studies in this area whilst clinical studies and depression treatment trials have also shown the same causal link (Lustman, et al., 2005; 2000a). The strong association between depression and the onset of Type 2 diabetes is therefore clearly indicated and conversely, those who already have diabetes are at an increased risk of developing depression due to effects of sustained hyperglycaemia on the body's chemical and hormonal balance. This relationship between depression and the onset of Type 2 diabetes may be due to inactivity and weight gain, influencing metabolic changes. As we have seen, many of the medications used to treat depression lead to weight gain and sedation, which could also contribute to the development of Type 2 diabetes.

Having depression influences decision-making and motivation surrounding all aspects of life, such as dietary behaviour, smoking, exercise, thought processes and participating in diabetes self-care activities requiring diligent, ongoing attention. Research by Ciechanowski, et al., (2003) and Lustman and Clouse, (2002) shows this to be the case. Almost 7 million people in the United Kingdom (Diabetes UK, 2017) and 88 million American adults have pre-diabetes (Center for Disease Control and Prevention, 2020), placing them at increased risk for developing Type 2 diabetes. Pre-diabetes is defined as blood glucose concentrations higher than normal, but lower than established thresholds for diabetes itself. Whilst not all cases of depression will ultimately lead to pre-diabetes, this significantly increases the risk of later developing Type 2 diabetes. There is also a causal link between having depressive episodes when younger – <30 years of age – and the accelerated onset of diabetes in at-risk individuals (Brown, et al., 2005).

The purpose of glucose self-monitoring is to regulate metabolic control, but certain physiological mechanisms cause hyperglycaemia when depression is also present, meaning regulation of insulin dosages or diabetes medication is impaired. Research in this area suggests that depression causes glucocorticoid disruption – the release of hormones such as cortisol in times of stress; an increase in the activity of the sympathetic nervous system – triggering the release of stored glucose from the liver, and alterations in the inflammatory process – all increasing HbA1c, exacerbating insulin resistance (Boden and Hoeldtke, 2003; Musselman, et al., 2003; Ramasubbu, 2002).

Insulin resistance – where the body cannot use insulin effectively – is the same as pre-diabetes and is a pre-cursor to the development of Type 2 diabetes. The link between insulin resistance and developing diabetes still requires further research as it is only a potential indicator that the condition may occur, although there is growing evidence suggesting that insulin resistance is due to depression. It has been shown for over 30 years that non-diabetic individuals with depression have increased blood glucose levels and a reduced insulin response during glucose tolerance testing (Timonen, et al., 2005).

Brown, et al. (2005) state that Type 2 diabetes may not be the only chronic health condition that develops following an episode of depression. This is very difficult to quantify, although preventative strategies could be put in place for these conditions. This is especially important for young individuals being treated for depression, highlighting that mental health problems should be regarded as a key risk factor for future chronic illness over genetic and lifestyle factors.

Similarly, Wax (2013) suggests that the hormones released during a period of stress and depression – cortisol and epinephrine – lower the immune system, reducing the release of serotonin, resulting in listless and joyless feelings. Wax states that if these hormone levels remain high they can lead to heart disease, hardening of the arteries, Type 2 diabetes, and certain cancers due to impaired immune system function. Chapman, et al. (2005) have also confirmed that depression undoubtedly leads to further chronic health conditions.

It is clear that depression affects the individual with diabetes by severely impairing their health-related quality of life, reducing physical activity levels, limiting concordance with diabetes self-care regimes, and by impairing the individual's ability to communicate effectively with health professionals. A treatment plan for depression should ideally be individually tailored to needs after a full assessment and should involve the individual's partner and key family members if appropriate. This is dependent on resources, however, and availability may vary widely from area to area. Both anti-depressant medication and psychotherapy are equally effective in treating depression and approximately 50–60 percent of patients will achieve remission within 3 months (Clark, 2004b).

Key messages in this chapter:

- Depression leads to significant consequences such as loss of employment, productivity and income.
- There is a 2 percent higher risk of death from all causes for individuals with depression compared to those without the condition.
- Depression negatively affects the reporting of any symptoms associated with diabetes to healthcare professionals and reduces the individual's concordance with medical advice and diabetes self-care behaviour, leading to poor glycaemic control.
- A number of physical and psychological changes occur in diabetes, causing neurochemical and neurovascular abnormalities that trigger depression; genetic factors also have a role.
- A sedentary lifestyle and obesity – the two main risk factors for the development of Type 2 diabetes – are also associated with depression.
- The diagnosis of major depressive disorder is made when the symptoms occur together, when they are severe, and when they persist daily for a minimum of two weeks. Despite this, depression in diabetes is recognised and treated in less than a third of individuals.
- As few as 40 percent of individuals with diabetes remain free of major depressive disorder in the year following successful initial treatment, with recurrence of symptoms frequently accompanied by a deterioration in glycemic control.
- Management guidelines only provide a framework for treating diabetes as the primary condition and not coexisting conditions such as depression.
- Both anti-depressant medication and psychotherapy are equally effective in treating depression and approximately 50–60 percent of patients will achieve remission within 3 months.
- Remaining on a recovery dose of treatment for depression despite an improvement in symptoms continues the improvement in order to prevent relapse.

5 Diabetes and Eating Disorders

The rapid weight loss in pre-diagnosed Type 1 diabetes is due to ketoacidosis, where the body burns fat and protein stores for fuel when glucose cannot be used in the lack of insulin.

Following a diagnosis of Type 1 diabetes, a diet and insulin routine is established to improve glycaemic control. Insulin induces hunger and lays down fat stores; any insulin dosage must also be 'fed' with a certain amount of carbohydrates to avoid low blood glucose levels, especially when exercising. This means it is more likely for adolescent females with Type 1 diabetes to have a higher body mass index than those without diabetes (Starkey and Wade, 2010; Larger, 2005). Weight gain is therefore brought about by successful insulin treatment, or rather, the weight lost pre-diagnosis is regained with additional fat stores. Weight gain may concern the individual, triggering action to halt or reverse this development, leading to disordered eating that may ultimately result in an eating disorder. For those with Type 2 diabetes, weight gain will increase the dosage of diabetes medication or insulin and, as a consequence, hunger and dietary intake.

Prevalence, diabetes, and disordered eating

Certain individuals with diabetes are more likely to have an eating disorder such as anorexia, bulimia, binging, purging, or dangerous dieting habits than members of the general public (Brown and Mehler, 2015; Hsu, et al., 2009; Mannucci, et al., 2005). For adolescents with Type 1 diabetes, risk of developing an eating disorder is two-and-a-half times greater than adolescents without the condition and this group is 16 times more likely to die from anorexia nervosa (Neilsen, et al., 2002). Diabetes UK (2017) state that 1 in every 50 individuals with Type 1 diabetes and 1 in 10 persons with Type 2 has an eating problem, the greater number

DOI: 10.4324/9781003260219-6

with Type 2 diabetes being responsible for its major prevalence. Disordered eating occurs more frequently in those with Type 1 diabetes.

> 'I basically binge eat when I'm unhappy. Then my blood glucose levels are really high. When I'm like that I don't stop to calculate, "crisps plus ice cream plus cake plus chocolate equals such and such carbohydrate units". It makes it hard to judge the right amount of insulin for all that I've eaten – I don't even know how much I've eaten!'
>
> 'Since I was 15, I've been taking less insulin than I should because it helps me lose weight. I've always lost about 6kg when I have bad ketoacidosis because of an infection and high sugar levels. Now I'm older, when I have to get weight down the temptation is always there to use that method rather than to alter my diet sensibly'.

Hypoglycaemia – low blood glucose levels – stimulates the hypothalamus to increase appetite so that blood glucose levels can be raised to protect the brain. Insulin pump therapy is prescribed in Type 1 diabetes, commonly due to the clinical need of frequent and unpredictable hypoglycaemia. The individual proactively uses this technology to achieve good glycaemic control, preventing/ameliorating complications. However, pump therapy may be used inappropriately, allowing predominantly young female patients to drastically reduce their insulin dosage – perhaps to avoid hypoglycaemia in the short-term – resulting in long-term hyperglycaemia and weight loss. Insulin pump therapy delivers a continual basal dose of short-acting insulin, with bolus amounts given to cover the carbohydrate content of meals and snacks. Disordered eating occurs where the background dose of insulin enables the individual to skip meals; this is more difficult to achieve with insulin injections. (Wilson, 2012).

Deliberate insulin under-dosing or omission is known as diabulimia – inducing drastic weight loss with hyperglycaemia, leading to ketoacidosis. This practice is common in females with diabetes (Young, et al., 2013), although a 5-year prospective study found that glycaemic control was unaffected by eating disorders (Colton, et al., 2007). However, marked fluctuations in blood glucose levels are inevitable when there is reduced insulin and over or under-eating. Therefore, a significant link exists between disordered eating and poor glycaemic control. This could be due to denial because diabetes is a condition dominated by dietary regulation and portion control, with great emphasis on the need for carbohydrate awareness as starches are broken down by the body for energy, increasing blood glucose levels.

Fear of hypoglycaemia

Hypoglycaemia is an acute side-effect of the temporary excess of diabetes medications – insulin and/or sulfonylureas – in the absence of sufficient blood glucose. If mild hypoglycaemia goes undetected and untreated, glucose continues to fall, resulting in severe hypoglycaemia, requiring the assistance of another person to treat it. Low blood glucose levels may be recurrent, causing extreme fear (Snoek, et al., 2000), especially for those taking insulin. This fear is not unfounded if severe hypoglycaemic episodes have previously occurred, leading to concern about being unconsciousness – especially in a public place where others do not understand what action to take; having an accident/injury; becoming emotionally upset or uncooperative, and/or creating an embarrassing situation. There is also the rare possibility that severe hypoglycaemia may lead to sudden death.

Research shows that fear of hypoglycaemia is more pronounced in adults with Type 1 diabetes and a history of severe hypoglycaemia. This is based on variables such as:

- loss of consciousness, especially during sleep, or hospitalisation
- frequent hypoglycaemia that impairs ability to work (Anderbro, et al., 2018)
- impaired awareness of hypoglycaemia (Gold, et al., 1994)

As some adults with Type 2 diabetes treat their condition with insulin, risk of hypoglycaemia is clearly increased. Hajós, et al (2014) found that taking insulin engendered a greater fear of hypoglycaemia than taking sulphonylurea medication – which can also increase the risk of low blood glucose levels. Prevalence of severe hypoglycaemia increases in adults with Type 2 diabetes using insulin for more than five years, meaning fear of hypoglycaemia is similar to adults with Type 1 diabetes; anticipation of problematic hypoglycaemia can be a psychological barrier to insulin initiation for those currently using oral diabetes medication (Diabetes UK, 2019).

'I was a health professional and couldn't afford a hypo while working in theatre or driving between hospitals as a locum – I didn't even tell my colleagues I had diabetes [Type 1]. I let my glucose levels run high to avoid hypos, knowing the complications risk. Now I'm retired with retinopathy and nerve damage as a result'.

'I've got Type 2 treated with insulin so occasionally, I go low and feel really shaky and bad-tempered. If I'm going out socially, I take less evening insulin and eat much more when I'm out because I don't want to feel unwell and miss out on the evening, especially not with other people around me'.

In addition to individual psychiatric predisposition, people with diabetes can be more susceptible to disordered eating behaviours because of the nature of this chronic condition (Peraira and Alvarenga, 2007). The prevalence of eating disorders in individuals with diabetes may be explained by the perception of body dissatisfaction, a desire to lose weight because of insulin-related weight gain, feelings of obsession with food, perception of lost control, the belief that diabetes governs life, and the experience of independence or dependence conflicts. However, the trigger for disordered eating is highly individual.

Research suggests that disordered eating behaviour develops when the individual tries to lose weight due to body dissatisfaction (Ackard, et al., 2008). An interesting phenomenon is the lack of desire to manage diabetes effectively coupled with wanting to stop diabetes exerting control over one's life or situation by restrictive eating and/or bulimia. Conditions like anorexia are rooted in the individual's desire to have control over their lives (Young-Hyman and Davis, 2010). A fear of hypoglycaemia and a desire to avoid low blood glucose levels may also lead the individual to take less insulin, especially when driving – risk aversion – or when working – aiming to avoid stigma and a desire not to draw attention.

The motivation for this rationalisation may be a wish to avoid the unpleasant side effects of hypoglycaemia and the lack of control hypoglycaemia exerts over the body at these times. This is especially the case if the individual is reliant on another person to administer something sweet, or give a glucagon injection if they fall unconscious with no hypoglycaemic warning signs. A fear of hypoglycaemia can also lead the individual to eat more to prevent low glucose levels, or to reduce insulin dosage so glucose levels are higher. Over time, this behaviour increases the risk of chronic complications of diabetes.

Disordered eating conditions

The terms disordered eating and eating disorders are not the same. Eating disorders refer to psychiatric disorders marked by disturbed eating behaviours, disordered food intake, disordered eating attitudes, and often inadequate methods of weight control. Disordered eating describes all eating-related problems, from a calorie-controlled diet to clinical eating disorders, such as anorexia nervosa and bulimia nervosa (American Psychiatric Association, 2006). It is essential for those with diabetes to obtain the right diagnosis of their eating condition as these disorders can significantly increase diabetes morbidity and mortality (Peraira and Alvarenga, 2007; Kelly, et al., 2005), as well as weight gain, poor metabolic control, insulin omission, and an increased prevalence of microvascular complications (Peraira and Alvarenga, 2007; Rydall, et al., 1997).

Anorexia

Anorexia nervosa is a severe psychological disorder describing an absent desire for food. The *Diagnostic and Statistical Manual Criteria of Mental Disorders* (DSM-5, American Psychiatric Association, 2013) classifies anorexia as a condition where there is an obsessive fear of gaining weight resulting in severe dietary restriction. The condition develops more frequently in young women than in the wider population. Concurrent Type 1 diabetes and anorexia nervosa is a rare but serious condition in females. All indexes of mortality evidence excess mortality (Nielsen, et al., 2002), making robust and well-directed treatment efforts essential for this subpopulation.

Collaboration between diabetes clinicians and eating disorder specialists is necessary. The implications of other eating disorders and subclinical eating disorders in diabetic populations have been reported more frequently, perhaps because these conditions are more numerous than clinical eating disorders.

Studies of young women with Type 1 diabetes have focused on the ages of 15–35 years, where there is a higher prevalence of eating disorders (Mannucci, et al., 2005), although Daneman, et al. (2002) suggests that adolescent girls and young women with Type 1 diabetes rarely experience anorexia nervosa. Further research has recognised that anorexia also occurs in other populations, such as males (Neumark-

Sztainer, et al., 2002) and individuals with Type 2 diabetes (Rodin, et al., 2002; Crow, et al., 2000).

Body dysmorphia and a distorted body image are common motivating triggers for anorexic behaviour. Individuals are often of normal weight or even underweight, but see themselves as being grossly overweight. Consequently, food dominates every aspect of the individual's life and they eat sparingly, weighing and calorie-counting everything to control their intake. This parallels the diabetes lifestyle to a large extent, so being taught and encouraged by healthcare professionals to be vigilant with diet can be taken to the extreme as it gives permission for this behaviour within the need for diabetes self-care. One young woman with both Type 1 diabetes and a history of anorexia nervosa described how she became obsessed with her dietary intake:

'I used to be a normal weight, but portion control and exercise were always emphasised to manage my diabetes. I hated the strictness of the condition and started cutting out more and more food until I was basically only eating about 400 calories a day. This meant I needed hardly any insulin and some days, I didn't take any at all because I figured I could exist on the glucose my body couldn't deal with. Eventually my weight dropped to 35 kilos and I was told my heart muscle was damaged. With help from the hospital dietician, I realised I was just slowly killing myself. There's no real control over anything in life, only the best you can do under the circumstances'.

In a 12-year follow-up of 14 women with Type 1 diabetes and anorexia nervosa by Walker, et al. (2002), the women were aged between 25–46 years with an average 26-year duration of diabetes. Five of the women died at the average age of 30 years: two were found dead at home having developed severe hypoglycaemia – both women had hypoglycaemia unawareness; another died as a result of deliberate insulin omission and the onset of prolonged ketoacidosis. One died of sudden respiratory arrest two days after bone graft surgery for a non-healing fracture; the fifth woman died from emaciation following severe autonomic neuropathy compromising her gastrointestinal system, causing continual diarrhoea and vomiting. These five deaths were avoidable and the coexistence of an eating disorder with Type 1 diabetes was fatal for these women. Ten of the women had actually recovered from anorexia nervosa and were of a normal BMI, demonstrating that the damage to their bodies was irreparable. Walker, et al. (2002) recorded a mortality rate of 36 percent over 12 years with a high rate of microvascular morbidity.

Individuals with eating disorders have a high prevalence of associated medical complications in contrast to other mental health conditions. A review of the specific complications associated with anorexia nervosa showed that medical complications are a direct result of weight loss and malnutrition (Mehler and Brown, 2015). As with diabetic ketoacidosis, complications occur when glucose cannot be used by the cells as fuel, because starvation induces protein and fat catabolism – chemical reactions that break down complex compounds with the release of energy – causing shrinkage of the cell and a loss of function. This damage leads to adverse effects, such as atrophy of the heart, brain, liver, intestines, kidneys, and muscles. Almost every body system can be adversely affected by this state of ongoing malnutrition (Löwe, et al., 2001). These effects include physiological complications such as hypotension, bradycardia, and hypothermia – a reduced core body temperature below 35 degrees centigrade.

More than half of all deaths in those with anorexia nervosa are due to medical complications (National Institute for Health and Clinical Excellence, 2004), many being the same or similar to the complications of diabetes resulting from poor glycaemic control. Löwe, et al., (2001) state that for individuals with anorexia alone, the death rate is 10–12 times greater than in the general population and greater still when the individual has Type 1 diabetes. The main risk factors for developing medical complications associated with anorexia nervosa are the degree of weight loss and the duration of the illness (Miller, et al., 2005). The addition of chronic poor glycaemic control with blood glucose levels >15 mmol/L or >270 mg/dl and episodes of diabetic ketoacidosis exerts extreme stress on the body, significantly altering metabolic parameters.

Complications of anorexia and diabetes

With poor nutrition causing further weight loss, individuals with anorexia commonly have dry skin which can split open and bleed, especially on the fingers and toes (Strumia, 2005). When anorexia and diabetes coexist, this is problematic due to slow wound healing associated with poor blood supply and nerve damage in 50 percent of people with diabetes. Individuals with anorexia are often intolerant to cold and have a bluish discoloration of their fingertips, nose and ears – acrocyanosis – due to maintaining blood flow to vital organs in response to hypothermia.

Poor blood flow to the extremities is common in those with diabetes due to microvascular damage, the process being amplified by the additional complications of anorexia nervosa (Gobel-Fabri, et al., 2008). Fine, downy hair on the sides of the face and along the spine – lanugo hair growth – is commonly experienced by individuals with anorexia nervosa; this may develop to conserve body heat when there are reduced fat deposits (Mehler and Brown, 2015). Ulcerated areas of skin covering bony prominences such as elbows and heels develop due to loss of supporting subcutaneous tissue; bruising also often occurs due to reduced subcutaneous tissue (Miller, et al., 2005).

When weight is reduced below approximately 15–20 percent of ideal body weight, there is often the development of gastroparesis (Kamal, et al., 1991). Gastroparesis describes delayed stomach emptying, causing bloating, early fullness, flatulence and upper quadrant pain. This condition is also associated with autonomic nerve damage in diabetes (Wilson, 2004a), resulting in slow digestive transit, with symptoms such as vomiting – relating to the upper gastrointestinal tract, and/or alternating constipation and diahorrea – relating to the lower GI tract. Constipation often occurs in individuals with anorexia nervosa due to slow transit in the colon when very little food is available to process, resulting in under-activity of the reflex of the colon (Mehler and Brown, 2015). In addition, gastrointestinal disorders such as irritable bowel syndrome are more common in those with anorexia than in the wider population (Porcelli, et al., 1998).

The liver normally produces enzymes – transaminases – to break down and synthesise amino acids, converting them into energy storage molecules. The two main enzymes – Alanine Transaminase (ALT) and Aspartate Transaminase (AST) – are usually low in concentration, but if there is liver damage, the outer membrane of the liver cells has greater permeability so these enzymes leak into the bloodstream. Enzyme leakage is abnormal in almost 50 percent of individuals with anorexia nervosa as weight loss and fasting leads to mildly elevated levels.

Marked enzyme elevation may be a sign of organ failure in severe anorexia (De Caprio, et al., 2006). Liver enzyme levels can also be mildly elevated if the individual with anorexia is hospitalised and fed with intravenous dextrose – a condition known as steatosis. This stabilises if calorie intake from dextrose is reduced temporarily and liver function improves with nutritional support. The liver shrinks in size when the body is forced into starvation mode and following dextrose infusion, the organ has a fatty appearance during ultrasound scanning, although the reason for this is unknown (Harris, et al., 2013).

Individuals with anorexia nervosa may also develop a condition known as superior mesenteric artery syndrome, where the duodenum becomes compacted between the aorta and the spine posteriorly and the superior mesenteric artery anteriorly. With an extreme loss of body fat, this narrows the angle of the blood vessels, trapping the duodenum (Mehler and Brown, 2015). The condition causes pain after eating, a feeling of early fullness, nausea and vomiting. Protein malnutrition in severe anorexia may lead to the inhalation of liquids and solids due to weakened pharyngeal muscles (Holmes, et al., 2012). Acute pancreatitis can also occur where pancreatic enzymes – trypsin, lipase and amylase – are activated and the pancreas becomes inflamed (Morris, et al., 2004). Acute pancreatitis can lead to diabetes as the insulin-producing cells of the pancreas are damaged by this inflammation. Each of these complications of anorexia significantly increases mortality risk in those with Type 1 diabetes.

Endocrine abnormalities associated with anorexia

Anorexia nervosa causes many problems with the endocrine system, compromising its function, including loss of bone density that may be associated with elevated cortisol levels (Lo Sauro, et al., 2008). There are also usually elevated levels of growth hormone (Mehler and Brown, 2015), although levels of insulin-like growth factor are reduced (Estour, et al., 2010). In some individuals with anorexia, low levels of anti-diuretic hormone may lead to diabetes insipidus – a rare condition affecting the pituitary gland, characterised by severe thirst and frequent urination, but this urine does not contain glucose.

Reduced thyroid function – hypothyroidism – is also common with anorexia, where thyroxin (T_4) and triiodothyronine (T_3) are low, decreasing with the degree of weight loss, although thyroid stimulating hormone (TSH) levels are usually normal (Utiger, 1995). With correct nutrition, these abnormalities are reversed, but thyroid hormone replacement medication is not recommended as it can cause reduced bone density and osteoporosis, this complication already being associated with anorexia (Mehler and Brown, 2015).

Severe weight loss and excessive exercise associated with anorexia nervosa results in hypoglycaemia and abnormal glucose metabolism of non-carbohydrate sources such as amino acids, glycerol or lactic acid. This process – gluconeogenesis – normally enables the release of glucose when required (Wilson, 2014). In advanced anorexia, there is no stored glucose when blood glucose falls below normal levels. Severe hypoglycaemia – <2 mmol/L or 36 mg/dl – in those with diabetes and/or anorexia can lead to death because the brain has insufficient glucose to continue heart and respiratory function. Sudden death from hypoglycaemia in those with anorexia is due to the depletion of glycogen to maintain normal blood glucose levels.

Insulin levels are reduced in non-diabetic individuals with anorexia when hypoglycaemia occurs, despite the condition being due to an excess of insulin. However, this counter-regulation may be lost after many years of anorexia (Tseng, et al., 2014), with a reduction in blood glucose levels due to the body producing too much insulin with intravenous feeding (Yashuhara, et al., 2003). Type 1 diabetes occasionally develops in those with anorexia nervosa, possibly due to the inflammation of insulin-producing pancreatic cells. As we have already seen, individuals with Type 1 diabetes may also develop anorexia, leading to treatment challenges and an increased mortality risk.

Eating disorders such as anorexia rarely occur in people with Type 2 diabetes (Young-Hyman and Davis, 2010). When individuals with Type 1 diabetes are treated for anorexia using structured feeding, a blood glucose level of no higher than 13.9mmol/L or 250mg/dl, is allowed in the shorter term as need for nutrition outweighs the long-term risk of chronic complications of diabetes. Once weight is restored, tight glycaemic control is the aim (Mehler and Brown, 2014).

Disruption to sex hormones due to anorexia nervosa is seen in both male and female individuals. Reduced levels of hypothalamic gonadotrophin releasing hormone – GnTR, pituitary luteinizing hormone – LH, follicle stimulating hormone – FSH, oestrogen and testosterone are seen, affecting fertility, potency and bone density (Mehler and Brown, 2015). A healthy reproductive cycle depends on the release of GnRH – gonadotrophin releasing hormone – to control levels of LH and FSH by the pituitary gland, determining menstruation. Females with anorexia experience absence of menstrual periods – hypothalamic amenorrhea syndrome – as hormonal disruption results in a failure to ovulate, although this is reversible – known as functional amenorrhea. Absence of menstruation may occur prior to significant weight loss in 20–25 percent of females with anorexia, while 50–75 percent experience amenorrhea whilst dieting (Dalle-Grave, et al., 2008).

Hormonal changes associated with anorexia reduce the chance of conception, although ovulation continues and pregnancy may occur despite absent menstruation (Bulik, et al., 2010). In females with diabetes, there is a higher risk of complications throughout pregnancy (Koubaa, et al., 2005), and a higher rate of miscarriage (Builk, et al.,

1999). When there is hormonal disruption during gestation, 18 percent of pregnant mothers develop gestational diabetes, occurring in the twentieth week of pregnancy; the condition is similar to Type 2 diabetes with high glucose levels. If the mother already has diabetes, the child is six times more likely to also develop diabetes at some point. With the addition of an eating disorder, developmental problems for the foetus are inevitable.

MRI brain scans of those with anorexia nervosa have shown brain shrinkage – atrophy, similar to those with Type 1 diabetes who have suffered repeated episodes of unconsciousness due to severe hypogly-caemia (Asvoid, et al., 2010; Ehrlich, et al, 2008). When severe, this damage is indistinguishable on an MRI scan from the appearance of Alzheimer's disease (Kraeft, et al., 2013). Weight gain in those with anorexia does not restore normal brain function; grey and white brain matter damage can be revealed on MRI scans associated with duration of the illness (Lazaro, et al., 2013). Research using positron emission to-mography scans aims to identify areas of the brain most affected during starvation in the hope of developing a treatment (Mehler and Brown, 2015). When there is long-term damage to the peripheral nerves in diabetes, the same damage does not occur in those with anorexia.

Bone marrow disorders are common in 75 percent of those with extreme weight loss, affecting the red and white blood cells and the platelets (Mehler and Brown, 2015; Sabel, et al., 2013). Anaemia and a low white blood cell count – leukopenia – is seen in around one-third of individuals with anorexia, and a low red blood cell count – thrombo-cytopenia – in ten percent, which may be associated with impaired liver function, (Sabel, et al., 2013). The appearance of bone marrow changes due to starvation, becoming gelatinous with a lack of fat because this has been leeched from the bone as a source of energy (Abella, et al., 2002). Unlike individuals with Type 1 diabetes and lowered immune system function, those with anorexia are not predisposed to infections, despite a reduced white cell count (Brown, et al. 2005).

Loss of bone volume – osteoporosis – or osteopenia – loss of bone density, occurs in 85 percent of women with anorexia, with prevalence of fractures being 60 percent higher than the non-anorexic population (Fazeli and Klibanski, 2014). Bone mass may never be normal if anorexia develops during adolescence as bone accumulation continues until the mid-twenties (Mehler and Brown, 2015). There is also reduced bone mineral density when compared to women who develop anorexia as adults where there is amenorrhea (Misra and Klibanski, 2014). Reduced testosterone affecting bone mineral density and osteoporosis in males with anorexia tends to be more significant than in females (Mehler, et al., 2008). Osteoporosis is seen in older individuals with diabetes as bone health is compromised by the condition; there is an increased risk of osteoporosis-related bone fractures in both Type 1 and Type 2 diabetes, especially to the hip joint (Brown and Sharpless, 2004).

A low bone mass is caused by reduced bone formation and increased bone reabsorption due to hormonal changes such as the elevated level of growth hormone during starvation. Insulin-like growth factor and growth hormone influence bone metabolism and ensure normal bone mass is maintained, although there is a deficiency in those with anorexia (Mehler and Brown, 2015). Similarly, in Type 1 diabetes there is reduced insulin-like growth factor (Jehle, et al., 1998).

Diabetes exerts a predisposition towards premature and enhanced small and large blood vessel disease. Anorexia also adversely affects cardiac function, causing low blood pressure – hypotension; while bradycardia – a slow sinus rhythm of less than 60 beats per minute – is seen in up to 95 percent of individuals (Mehler and Brown, 2015). Low blood pressure and heart rate return to normal with correct nutrition and weight gain (Ulger, et al., 2006). Abnormalities in the structure of the heart are also common in anorexia, with a collection of fluid in the pericardial sac surrounding the heart – pericardial effusion – seen in 70 percent of individuals (Kastner, et al., 2012; Doxc, et al., 2010). This may be due to rapid weight loss and low T_3 and insulin-like growth factor; both of which are usually reversed with weight gain (Inagaki, et al., 2003).

Additional problems, such as decreased ventricular mass, decreased cardiac output, and decreased systolic and diastolic dimensions, have been reported (Kastner, et al., 2012). Similar problems experienced by those with anorexia have been reported in diabetes, with pericardial effusion seen in adolescents with Type 1 diabetes (Koronouri, et al., 2009). Reduced cardiac output in diabetes has been reported by Pop-Busui (2010), as have systolic and diastolic abnormalities (Höke, et al., 2013).

Air in the pleural space causes lung collapse – pneumothorax, while tension pneumothorax describes the development of a valve allowing air into the pleural space which cannot escape, pushing the heart, lungs, trachea, oesophagus and other structures towards the unaffected lung. These are a relatively rare complication of anorexia nervosa, but both conditions present a medical emergency (Biffl, et al., 2014). Cases of spontaneous tension pneumothorax and pneumoperineum – air in the abdominal cavity – develop due to self-induced vomiting, causing acute gastric rupture in individuals who starve and purge themselves (Mehler and Brown, 2015). Tension pneumothorax has been documented in those with Type 1 diabetes and severe ketoacidosis (Steenkamp, et al., 2011).

Ketoacidosis

Anorexia nervosa and diabetes mellitus share similar complications – protein breakdown in ketoacidosis as an alternative source of fuel for the body is common to both conditions. In diabetes, glucose cannot be used for fuel in the lack of insulin and with anorexia, insufficient carbohydrates, proteins and fats are consumed so the body has to break down muscle protein for fuel. Both of these situations present a serious medical emergency.

Males with anorexia are at higher risk of developing ketoacidosis than females because they generally have a lower percentage of body fat and a greater lean muscle mass; males of all ages who suffer from disordered eating perceive and face stigma because anorexia is seen as a condition predominantly affecting females, meaning that they may postpone seeking treatment. For this reason, males with anorexia tend to have more pronounced weight loss and wide-ranging complications when they finally receive medical attention (Sabel, et al., 2014). Anorexia in males is associated with a reduced libido and shrunken testes, reduced testosterone, luteinising hormone and follicle stimulating hormone levels. Complications affecting every body system grow more severe with continued weight loss and starvation (Mehler and Brown, 2015), although unlike the chronic complications of diabetes – which can only be delayed with good glycaemic control – most complications of anorexia can be completely reversed with correct nutrition.

Bulimia nervosa

The *Diagnostic and Statistical Manual of Mental Disorders* describes bulimia and anorexia as both eating disorders and disordered eating behaviours (American Psychiatric Association, 2013). Bulimia shares many features with anorexia and some individuals alternate between these conditions. Bulimia describes binge eating episodes followed by self-induced vomiting and laxative abuse – purging behaviours – occurring at least twice a week for a period of three months due to perception of an abnormal body shape and weight. Bulimia nervosa may be classed as either purging or non-purging. The purging type involves regularly engaging in purging behavior, including self-induced vomiting or the abuse of laxatives, diuretics or enemas; the non-purging type describes compensatory behavior to prevent weight gain, such as fasting or excessive exercise (Criego, et al., 2009).

Eating behaviours affecting those with and without diabetes fall into a broad spectrum of disorders with clinical significance, although they do not meet the full diagnostic criteria for anorexia nervosa or bulimia nervosa. These include binge eating disorder; variants of bulimia nervosa where binge eating and purging occur less frequently than twice a week or where there is purging after eating normal amounts of food, and variants of anorexia nervosa – for example, where a three-month duration of amenorrhea is not present or where significant weight loss has occurred but bodyweight remains above 85 percent of expected weight (Criego, et al., 2009).

There are more moderate sub-categories of each of these behaviours that do not meet full *DSM of Mental Disorders* criteria, but still represent a significant health risk. As with full-blown eating disorders, these eating behaviours also necessitate clinical attention, particularly for those with Type 1 diabetes where disordered eating tends to be ongoing (Colton, et al., 2007). It is also known that anorexia may develop following a period of bulimic behaviour and that clinical bulimia nervosa is prevalent in Type 1 diabetic females (Mannucci et al., 2005; Schwartz, et al., 2000).

Among individuals with Type 1 diabetes, 27 percent of adolescents with bulimia use purgative practices, and 24 percent restrict their diets in an effort to lose weight (Pinhas-Hamlet and Levy-Shraga, 2013). Having diabetes increases the likelihood of developing disordered eating behaviours because of the necessity for precise meal planning and weighing of food portions, counting of carbohydrate values, the psychosocial issues associated with having diabetes, and the need for regular self-monitoring of the condition. Peraira and Alvarenga (2007) suggest that diagnosing disordered eating conditions such as anorexia and bulimia in the diabetes population is complicated by these factors.

It is estimated that one in every 400 children and adolescents and 11.8 percent of adult men and women has some form of bulimia nervosa, the condition being more prevalent in women with Type 1 diabetes (National Eating Disorders Association, 2021). Compulsive eating more than twice a week, followed by purges to get rid of the food – binge-eating disorder – is more prevalent in women with Type 2 diabetes (Centre for Disease Control and Prevention, 2011).

As with non-acceptance of the need for diabetes self-care activities, denial of disorderly eating behaviour is common, although studies featuring the individual's perspective are scarce. The National Eating Disorder Association estimates that 10 million females and one million males in the United States suffer from bulimia or anorexia, and that millions more struggle to manage binge-eating disorder (Morrison, 2012). Anorexia and bulimia share a number of physical complications, made worse by the addition of Type 1 diabetes.

'Taking insulin makes you fat. I ate properly in front of my parents, making myself sick a few times after meals, then I did it more and more. My parents noticed I was getting thinner and took me to the doctor, but I didn't let go of my secret. The doctor just suggested I eat more, telling me to speak to my diabetes consultant about the weight loss. No one realised it was bulimia for years because I'd had frequent diabetic ketoacidosis. As an adult, my teeth are crumbling from being sick so many times – stomach acid has eroded them. I also have heart problems – the doctors think that's due to high glucose levels, but I know better. In the end, I read in a book that if you put everything you ate in a day into a bucket it would look so horrible, why would you want to throw that up? Although I'm now 27 and I know it was a stupid thing to do, I'm also amazed that no one ever found out what I was hiding'.

Calorie restriction

When fasting leads to a shortage of food for energy and blood glucose levels drop, the liver uses its stores of glycogen to return glucose to the blood; energy stores can also be used in this way during vigorous exercise. Many individuals with diabetes fast periodically for religious reasons rather than because they have an eating disorder or a desire to lose weight. Religious fasts rarely exceed 24 hours (Al-Arouj, et al., 2010), although this practice leads to physiological changes as the body attempts to fuel the cells with a reduced amount of available energy.

Moving from eating to brief fasting and into prolonged starvation involves a series of metabolic, hormonal, and glucoregulatory mechanisms divided into three stages: the post-absorptive phase occurring 6–24 hours after commencing the fast; the gluconeogenic phase, from 2–10 days of fasting, and the protein conservation phase beyond 10 days of fasting (Felig, 1979). Fasting is a high-risk behaviour for individuals with Type 1 diabetes (Reiter, et al., 2007). This risk is heightened when there is poor diabetes control and limited access to medical care, hypoglycemic unawareness, unstable glycemic control, or recurrent hospitalisations.

The risk associated with fasting is much lower for individuals with Type 2 diabetes who manage their condition with diet and exercise alone (Uysal, et al., 1998), although there is still a potential risk of post prandial hyperglycemia once the fast is broken. If the individual takes diabetes medication to increase insulin sensitivity, the risk of hypoglycaemia during fasting is lower than with medications that increase insulin secretion – with the former, insulin is not produced in response to eating. If no food is consumed, the risk of hypoglycaemia for those taking Metformin to treat their Type 2 diabetes is also low, although dosage may need to be reduced (Mafauzy, et al., 1990).

A group of Type 2 diabetes medications are known as sulfonylureas – Chlorpromadine, Glibenclamide, Gliclazide, Gliciazide MR, and Nateglinide. These should not be taken when fasting because of the increased risk of hypoglycaemia, although if this does occur, it is unlikely to be as severe as in Type 1 diabetes (UK Prospective Diabetes Study – UKPDS, 1998a). Chlorpromadine may, however, cause unpredictable and prolonged hypoglycaemia if taken without food (Al-Arouj, et al., 2010), and Glyburide – also known as Glibenclamide – has an increased risk of hypoglycaemia compared with other sulfonylurea medications (Schernthaner, et al., 2004; Rendell, 2004).

Type 2 diabetes medications known as glitazones – Pioglitazone and Rosiglitazone – do not cause hypoglycaemia during fasting, although they can accelerate the blood glucose-lowering properties of sulfonylurea and glinides diabetes medication and insulin, if taken together (Mafauzy, et al., 1990). Weight gain is a common side-effect of glitazones, as well as increased appetite (Al-Arouj, et al., 2010), making fasting for the purpose of weight loss difficult to achieve. Additionally, glitazones take 2–4 weeks to have any substantial blood glucose management effect, so there is no association between hypoglycemia and fasting during this period (Retnakaran and Zinman, 2009).

Medications known as incretin-based therapy increase the effect of sulfonylureas, glinides and insulin: these are named Exenatide, Liraglutide, Dipeptidase-4 inhibitor, Alogliptin, Saxapliptin, Sitagliptin and Vildagliptin. Exenatide reduces feelings of hunger and stimulates weight loss, significantly affecting fasting blood glucose levels (Al-Arouj, et al., 2010).

Dipeptidase-4 is less effective at reducing blood glucose levels, although studies have suggested that they should be prescribed instead of sulfonylureas as they have fewer side-effects; the effects have not been studied during fasting (Drucker, 2010). Glucosidase inhibitor medications such as Acarbose, Miglitol and Voglibose are prescribed to slow down the rate of carbohydrate absorption; they exert little effect on fasting glucose and are not associated with an increased risk of hypoglycaemia when fasting (Al-Arouj, et al., 2010; Van de Laar, et al., 2005).

Insulin may be prescribed to manage Type 2 diabetes when medication becomes less effective in controlling hyperglycaemia. Short-acting insulins such as Repaglinide and Nateglinide may be used during fasting, but insulin lowers blood glucose levels and without food, this may lead to hypoglycaemia. During Ramadan, Mafauzy, et al. (1990) suggest that Repaglinide is less likely to cause hypoglycaemia than Glibenclamide. Of the sulfonylurea medications available, Natenglinide has the shortest working time and a lower risk of hypoglycaemia when fasting (Al-Arouj, et al., 2010). The incidence of fasting hypoglycaemia for those with Type 2 diabetes taking insulin is less than for those with Type 1 diabetes, the aim being prevention of fasting hypoglycaemia; insulin cannot be omitted when fasting as glucose levels must still be managed. The risk of hypoglycaemia when taking insulin is always present, especially when insulin has been prescribed for a number of years or if the individual is elderly with a higher risk of hypoglycaemia (Azizi, 2005).

As we have already seen, insulin pump therapy is a medical device predominantly used to deliver insulin in Type 1 diabetes, although some with Type 2 also use this method; pump therapy provides continuous subcutaneous insulin infusion with a cannula placed under the skin, mimicking the physiological action of the body as closely as possible. This is an intensive diabetes management technology and the pump user must learn how to vary the amount of insulin required at different times of the day and night, diligently using this method to achieve good glycaemic control. Blood glucose concentration changes constantly according to physiological factors, such as the rate at which food is digested and the type of food eaten; planned and unplanned exercise; stress and emotional upset, and illness (Wilson, 2005).

Fasting can be undertaken when using pump therapy, with frequent self-monitoring of blood glucose to manage glucose levels without food. This is possible because pump therapy delivers an ongoing background dose of insulin to maintain glucose levels and can be programmed to deliver a bolus of insulin when needed for food. The pump user determines basal insulin requirements throughout the day and night by monitoring peaks and troughs in glucose levels with finger prick blood tests. Pump therapy offers the opportunity of fasting with less risk of hypoglycaemia, but only if insulin and blood glucose levels are correctly calculated. As we have seen, some individuals with Type 1 diabetes have taken advantage of this insulin delivery system to maintain anorexic and bulimic behaviours (Badescu, et al., 2016).

Diabulimia

When both diabetes and disordered eating coexist, it has often been referred to as diabulimia – also known as ED-DMT1 (eating disorder-diabetes mellitus Type 1) in the US, or T1ED (Type 1 eating disorder) in the UK, although this terminology does not properly address all types of disordered eating patterns. Diabulimia is serious, but it is not a recognised mental illness in its own right (Diabetes UK, 2018). For individuals with Type 1 diabetes, omitting or drastically reducing insulin dosages for the purpose of achieving weight loss actually falls under the category of bulimia nervosa in the general category of purging behaviour.

Diabulimia is a persistent and distressing condition, largely unrecognised by the medical profession, perhaps because this term was coined by individuals with Type 1 diabetes to describe the condition; diabulimia only affects those with Type 1 diabetes and people with Type 2 cannot develop diabulimia (Diabetes UK, 2018). The condition is cited in the literature as disordered eating rather than as an eating disorder in its own right in the context of adolescent females with Type 1 diabetes.

Diabulimia has been a recognised problem since the 1980s, although there is no diabetes-specific measure of the condition, making prevalence or the psychological effects of diabulimia difficult to assess. Eating disorders generally occur less frequently in young males than they do in young females, calculated at one in every 400 males, compared with 1 in 50 females (NICE, 2004). Because eating disorders are less common in young males than in young females with Type 1 diabetes, diabulimia is even rarer in diabetic males. Diabetes UK (2018) state that the exact number living with diabulimia is unknown; it is estimated that around 4 out of 10 women, aged 15–30, take less insulin to lose weight and for young men, it is around 1 out of 10.

Assessing the rate of diabulimia largely relies on self-reporting. Available figures show that prevalence may be higher when applying the criteria for bulimia nervosa, including binge eating disorder (Young et al., 2013; Smith et al., 2008; NICE, 2004). Peveler, et al. (2005) suggest that prevalence ranges from 15–37 percent in adults – consistent with the National Eating Disorders Association (2021). This behaviour may be accompanied by binge eating, bulimia and excessive exercise – which can induce hyperglycaemia when there is insufficient insulin – by more young females suffering with Type 1 diabetes, shown to be eight percent when compared with one percent of non-diabetic girls (Colton et al., 2004).

Diabulimia behaviour

When an individual with Type 1 diabetes deliberately induces life-threatening ketoacidosis by restricting their insulin dosages, some factors make this behaviour more likely, such as the need for some form of control over life and bodyweight. Reduced insulin dosages may also be connected with the fear of severe hypoglycaemia. Extremely low blood glucose levels can be very frightening as the individual feels that they are unable to physically and mentally control what is happening to them, and they must rely on another person for a glucagon injection when unconscious, or something sweet to eat or drink if still conscious, if the individual cannot help themselves (Wilson, 2014). Significant cognitive dysfunction is associated with severe hypoglycaemia (Asvoid, et a., 2010; Auer, 2004).

As we have seen, diabulimia is common in female adolescents wishing to control their weight. Further factors known to make insulin-restricting behaviour more likely are weight gain following commencement of insulin treatment for Type 1 diabetes, where insulin stimulates hunger; low self-esteem accompanying the diagnosis of a chronic disease, highlighting that the adolescent is different from their peers; and any dysfunction within the family setting where major adjustments are made to accommodate the high demands of newly-diagnosed Type 1 diabetes into family routine.

Having diabetes means constant evaluation of what should and should not be eaten. Diabulimia is therefore a means of controlling both weight and the condition imposing these restrictions, although the behaviour eventually has negative consequences. For this reason, diabulimia is usually practised in secret over a period of time rather than being confined to one or two incidences of deliberately restricting insulin dosage; longitudinal studies suggest that diabulimia can become a chronic condition (Goebel-Fabri, 2008; Colton et al., 2007). Neumark-Sztainer (2002) showed that both women and men with Type 1 diabetes regarded regular insulin under-dosing as the most favoured method of weight control.

'I've been cutting down on my insulin to reduce weight for at least 35 years. It's always been my secret and I never told friends or my parents. Blood sugars only got out of control three times, so I had to go into hospital with ketosis. I'm quite proud of that, although I've got some eye and nerve problems. Worth it to stay slim though'.

'I was diagnosed with Type 1 as a young lad in the 1970s; I was quite plump and used to get teased. The diabetes made me thinner at first and I was accepted more. When my sugars were stabilised with insulin, the weight came back as I was supposed to eat three main meals with cereal, bread and potatoes or pasta and three snacks of plain biscuits, morning, afternoon and before bed every day. I started cutting back on the food and having less insulin. In those days, there were only urine tests for sugar levels, so I did what I could to keep the weight off. My levels must have been sky-high, and I carried on with this for almost 20 years. Now I know the damage I've done to my body'.

To determine why diabulimia occurs, Markowitz, et al. (2010) asked adolescent females with Type 1 diabetes if they had ever been overweight. The researchers concluded that this was the most likely reason to deliberately restrict insulin dosage to induce hyperglycaemia and ketoacidosis. Additionally, Svenson, et al. (2003) showed that adolescent males with Type 1 diabetes were likely to have a higher BMI than non-diabetic males. Starkey and Wade (2010) suggest adolescent females with Type 1 diabetes are more likely to have a higher body mass index than those without diabetes. This occurs because insulin lays down fat stores and induces hunger; the insulin dosage must also be 'fed' with a certain amount of carbohydrates to avoid low blood glucose levels, especially when exercising. A history of weight problems in the younger female population with Type I diabetes has been highlighted as the strongest indicator for omitting insulin to achieve weight control.

Bodyweight is a continual focus for health professionals and this can lead to weight concerns for people with either Type 1 or Type 2 diabetes if excess weight is perceived as a criticism. This is especially relevant for adolescent females with low self-esteem who are highly aware of their body image and how others see them. Young women with Type 1 diabetes and disordered eating behaviour have fewer positive attitudes and a lower level of self-esteem compared with their non-diabetic contemporaries.

Diabulimia diagnosis

A review of studies published over the last 25 years on the prevalence of eating disorders and insulin restriction among people with diabetes shows that 30–35 percent of women restrict insulin in order to lose weight at some point in their life. This number has remained relatively constant over the decades (National Eating Disorders Association, 2021). In a more recent study, one-third of female patients and one-sixth of male patients with Type 1 diabetes reported disordered eating and frequent insulin restriction (Wisting, et al., 2015).

The opportunity to diagnose diabulimia may be missed in primary care if there is not a high level of suspicion and specific questioning regarding this behaviour (Criego, et al., 2009). Diabetes healthcare professionals quickly recognise non-concordant diabetes self-care behaviours to determine why an individual might have poor glycaemic control. These signs include absence of finger-prick marks indicating a lack of regular SMBG and diabetes self-management behaviour; infrequent prescription requests for insulin or blood glucose testing strips; weight loss, or fluctuating bodyweight; erratic HbA1c measurements; mood changes and depressive behaviour. However, the healthcare professional has to know the individual well enough to recognise any of these changes. This presents a problem if health professionals are not visited on a regular basis, and if there is a high turnover of staff.

Diabulimia complications

Research into diabulimia has followed up the long-term outcome of this condition at eight and 12–year intervals (Goebel-Fabri, et al., 2008; Colton et al., 2007; Colton et al., 2004). Dangerous under-dosing of insulin and associated hyperglycaemia over a number of years resulted in the development of peripheral neuropathy, a complex condition affecting the feet and hands; peripheral neuropathy is a chronic complication of diabetes. This condition has two types: diffuse neuropathy, appearing as disorders of sensation in the extremities of the body; and distal polyneuropathy, affecting many nerves of the hands and feet. Restricting insulin to lose weight tripled the incidence of death (Goebel-Fabri et al., 2008).

Disordered eating and diabetes

For individuals with Type 1 or Type 2 diabetes, disordered eating induces behaviours that have cognitive, emotional and social consequences (Morrison, 2012). The cognitive impact of disordered eating leads to an obsession with food and eating; poor concentration and decision-making ability; disinterest in other activities; a distorted view of food and body image; denial; self-blaming; personalisation, and a tendency for over-generalisation. Emotional consequences include: depression and anxiety; irritability; guilt and shame; embarrassment; hopelessness; fear that the secret will be discovered; self-disgust after eating; low self-esteem, and a perceived loss of control. There are also social consequences as disordered eating leads to withdrawal from society, such as isolation; insecurity; mistrust of self and others, and a decreased or absent libido. It has been reported that some individuals spend a lot of money on binge foods, laxatives and diet pills, or that they shop-lift these items (Morrison, 2012).

As we have seen, those with diabetes and disordered eating behaviour are more likely to overlook the importance of diabetes self-care, for example, not carrying out regular SMBG. If the short-term consequences of poor diabetes control and high blood glucose levels are ignored, ketosis can develop. It is also the case that the long-term implications of prolonged poor control and the development or worsening of chronic complications are disregarded (Wilson, 2004b). Overall desire to be thin supersedes the pain and discomfort of dehydration and exhaustion during ketoacidosis, as well as the cognitive impairment associated with poor nutrition. Although restrictive eating is rare in someone with Type 2 diabetes as this condition is due in 90 percent of cases to obesity, the individual's diabetes may actually be reversed or drastically improved by restricted eating.

Binge eating without the correct dosage of insulin needed for the amount of food and drink consumed leads to hyperglycaemia and contributes to the development or worsening of complications. Weight gain due to binging is associated with health risks such as hypertension; hyperlipidaemia; increased fat stores around the organs, and sleep apnoea – excess fat around the neck which impairs breathing while the individual sleeps. Sleep apnoea has been associated with the development of Type 2 diabetes due to the effect of disrupted sleep on the immune system (Wax, 2013).

Treatment

Treating eating disorders and disordered eating in an individual who also has diabetes is challenging, requiring a collaborative approach between the diabetes team, the hospital dietician, and a clinical psychologist. These specialists aim to determine the cause of the disordered eating and work together to correct the behavior. The individual receives nutrition education that does not count carbohydrate, fat or calorie values, as well as learning to recognise health foods as beneficial to their diabetes. In this way, the individual moves away from an obsession with this aspect of food and towards correcting the eating disorder. The individual also learns how to monitor their weight normally (Bermudez and Sommer, 2012).

One of the greatest challenges in treating disordered eating and diabetes is the psychological impact of the condition; health professionals must be non-judgemental about the individual's health beliefs and behaviour. A clinical psychologist may not be available as many diabetes teams across the UK have no standard access to psychological support. A diabetes educator with specialist knowledge of eating disorders may then begin working with the individual (Morrison, 2012). The overall goal of the multi-disciplinary team is to improve metabolic control, reversing malnutrition and extreme weigh loss. It is usual for a parent or spouse of the diabulimic individual to take over insulin administration and blood glucose monitoring, or if the individual is a pump user, to return to injections (Herrin, 2003), although this clearly conflicts with a feeling of not being in control. Additionally, there is usually a clinical need for pump use when good glycaemic control cannot be achieved with injections. The perception of a person with Type 1 diabetes after beginning this type of counselling is seen below.

'I have a snack rather than a proper meal. I often eat because I'm bored or depressed and not because I'm hungry – eating loads of bad things because I'd already been bad and not given myself any extra insulin. After time spent with a counsellor and dietician, I can see that my binging and diabulimia is because I feel unhappy, defiant, depressed and hopeless and I want some form of control over my life. I've learned to really think about what I eat and the right insulin dosages by keeping a food diary'.

Over time the individual develops an improved relationship with food and does not associate eating with being a bad person, or regard ketoacidosis as a way to lose weight and be in control. Counselling emphasises that a choice is made about what is eaten. In this way, the individual gradually alters their perception of food. Eating disorders are therefore psychological diagnoses with physical complications (Morrison, 2012).

Key messages in this chapter:

- Anorexia nervosa is a severe psychological disorder describing an absent desire for food; it is an obsessive fear of gaining weight resulting in severe dietary restriction.
- Eating disorders such as anorexia rarely occur in people with Type 2 diabetes.
- Bulimia and anorexia are classed as both eating disorders and disordered eating behaviours.
- It is more likely for adolescents with Type 1 diabetes to have a higher body mass index than those without diabetes.
- For adolescents with Type 1 diabetes, risk of developing an eating disorder is two-and-a-half times greater than adolescents without the condition, and this group is 16 times more likely to die from anorexia.
- A significant link exists between disordered eating and poor glycaemic control. The association between diabetes and eating disorders may be explained by the perception of body dissatisfaction; a desire to lose weight because of insulin-related weight gain; feelings of obsession with food; perception of lost control; the belief that diabetes governs life, and having independence or dependence conflicts.
- Disordered eating and eating disorders are not the same. Eating disorders are psychiatric disorders marked by disturbed eating behaviours, disordered food intake, disordered eating attitudes, and often inadequate methods of weight control. Disordered eating describes all eating-related problems, from a calorie-controlled diet to clinical eating disorders, such as anorexia nervosa and bulimia nervosa.
- The main risk factors for developing medical complications associated with anorexia nervosa are degree of weight loss and duration of the illness. The addition of chronic poor glycaemic control, with blood glucose levels >15 mmol/L – >270 mg/dl in the USA, and episodes of diabetic ketoacidosis exert extreme stress on the body, significantly altering metabolic parameters.

- Bulimia nervosa may be classed as either purging or non-purging. The purging type involves regularly engaging in purging behavior, including self-induced vomiting or the abuse of laxatives, diuretics or enemas; the non-purging type describes compensatory behavior to prevent weight gain, such as fasting or excessive exercise.
- Compulsive eating behaviour more than twice a week, followed by purges to get rid of the food – binge-eating disorder – is more prevalent in women with Type 2 diabetes.
- Diabulimia – omitting or drastically reducing insulin dosages for the purpose of achieving weight loss – is classed under bulimia nervosa in the general category of purging behaviour rather than as a condition in its own right.
- Treating eating disorders and disordered eating in an individual who also has diabetes is challenging, requiring a collaborative approach between the diabetes team, the hospital dietician, and a clinical psychologist.

6   Diabetes and the Disease Process

Living well with diabetes requires good medical care and effective self-management skills. As we have seen, this is not possible without the individual's full engagement in their diabetes self-care; when Type 1 diabetes is very difficult to control; or when fighting an infection – where insulin requirements may increase threefold. Because continual fluctuations in blood glucose levels must be managed as well as possible, Type 1 or Type 2 diabetes exerts huge psychological demands on the individual. Even when blood glucose levels are well-managed, the nature of the condition and the impairment in metabolic function often heralds the onset of complications after a long duration of diabetes (Barnett and Grice, 2011). Proactive diabetes self-management may therefore only delay or reduce the severity of this eventual onset.

Chronic complications of diabetes

Chronic complications are the most common health problems for those with diabetes that are not a result of autoimmune disease. Elevated and prolonged blood glucose levels prior to diagnosis of Type 1 or Type 2 diabetes – or poor control of glucose levels after diagnosis – triggers the onset of these secondary, severe complications over time, such as nephropathy and retinal disease, neuropathy, cerebrovascular and heart disease. In general, every HbA1c percentage point reduction can reduce the risk of microvascular complications by 40 percent (Stratton, et al., 2000; Diabetes Control and Complications Trial Research Group, 1993). Annual eye and foot examination can reduce vision loss and lower-extremity amputations for those with diabetes. Identifying and treating diabetic retinopathy with laser therapy can halt the progression of severe vision loss by an estimated 50–60 percent (Kung, et al., 2008), while comprehensive foot care information and patient education can

DOI: 10.4324/9781003260219-7

lower amputation rates by 45–85 percent (MacRury, et al., 2018; Schofield, et al., 2009).

The high prevalence of chronic complications may be due to the difficulty in achieving near-normal HbA1c levels. A prevalence of complications in Type 2 diabetes study showed that of 66,726 people, 27.2 percent had macrovascular complications, while 53.5 percent had microvascular complications (Litwak, et al., 2013). Sun, et al. (2011) found that of 351 people with Type 1 diabetes with an average 50-year duration, 57.4 percent had proliferative retinopathy; 13.1 percent had nephropathy; 60.6 percent had neuropathy and 48.5 percent had cardiovascular disease. Despite the high prevalence of complications, little research has been published concerning the psychological impact for the individual: The vast majority of papers focus on good diabetes self-management to prevent the development of physical complications. Developing complications often leads to a victim blaming situation.

'I went to an appointment to have a mole removed. The dermatologist looked at my medical history, commenting that I obviously hadn't looked after my diabetes, as my eye and nerve problems were due to poorly-managed glucose levels. I pointed out that I'd had a lot of infections as a child, causing ketoacidosis that triggered the complications, but the dermatologist retained her blaming demeanour'.

'I saw an orthopaedic surgeon for a bone graft to my ankle after a break had left me with a shortened right tibia. He went on and on about my diabetes being badly managed because, after 40 years with Type 1 diabetes, I had very mild retinopathy – to be expected after such a long time with diabetes. He said the shortened limb was my fault. I was astonished and still think about being blamed years later'.

Prolonged and untreated hyperglycaemia undoubtedly triggers the onset of diabetic complications. However, some degree of complications eventually occurs due to ongoing abnormal levels of glucose in the cells, which is toxic and cannot be dealt with effectively. When glucose is metabolised by the body and energy is produced, carbon dioxide and water are released. High amounts of glucose impair the function of cells, so it is metabolised into sorbitol (Barnett and Grice, 2011). This substance accumulates in body tissues, causing damage as the fluid balance inside and outside the cells is equalised; these large sorbitol molecules cannot pass through the cell membrane and become trapped, resulting in damage and death of body cells. This metabolic imbalance and continual excessive glucose is a significant factor in the development of chronic complications. There may also be a genetic component, even when blood glucose levels are well-maintained (Barnett and Grice, 2011).

Although chronic complications frequently occur in those with long-duration diabetes due to altered metabolic parameters, and complications can still develop in those with well-controlled diabetes, coping with this additional disability is very much under-documented. Once complications are present they may be ameliorated with tighter glycaemic control, but they cannot be completely reversed; thus, prevention of complications has rightly been the focus of research. The individual's perspective following the development of complications requires investigation, as this additional poor health has both physical and psychological consequences.

'I've got Type 2 diabetes and have had two heart attacks. Doctors and nurses say it's my own fault because of my high blood sugars. Now I'm not at the prevention stage for complications, I just think I've been left on the scrap heap'.

'Since I was a baby I've had Type 1 diabetes and, 41 years on, there's some retinopathy and nerve damage. My diabetes consultant congratulated me for only having mild complications after such a long time, but other hospital staff seem to blame me. I have learned to live with my prickling feet and mild deterioration in sight because it happened gradually and I just got used to it, but hospital staff haven't offered psychological help'.

'A couple of years ago, I woke one day and I was blind. It took a long time to accept there was nothing I could do about it – although I still haven't really: diabetes has robbed me of my sight. I was given practical help – white stick, guide dog, taught braille etc., but no emotional help. I'm angry this has happened, hate myself for not taking better care when I had the chance, and bitter because I've lost a job I loved. I get that it takes time to adjust, but I'm stuck at being angry and bitter and I'm not the same person'.

'I've got autonomic nerve damage following repeated ketoacidosis as a child. It's affected my digestive system and I have delayed stomach emptying. Trying to give myself the right insulin to match rate of digestion is very hit and miss with lots of hypos and hypers. There's nothing I can do so I get very depressed. I've contemplated suicide several times, but that wouldn't be fair on my children, so I can't bring myself to go through with it. I just have to live with this nightmare that even my diabetes consultant doesn't understand because I don't have the same symptoms as other people'.

A fear of developing complications

With so much at stake for the individual, there is little doubt that people with either Type 1 or Type 2 diabetes are fearful of developing chronic complications (Speight, et al., 2001; Snoek, et al., 2000). This is especially the case when there is an increased risk of developing or worsening chronic complications due to prolonged, elevated glucose levels. However, research has found that this risk is often overestimated by the individual, leading to an increased fear of complications (Asimakopoulou, et al., 2008; Meltzer and Egleston, 2000). Increased emotional distress, anxiety and depression is correlated with worry about complications (Singh, et al., 2014; Meltzer, et al., 2000).

Diabetes health education strongly emphasises reducing the risk of long-term complications with good glycaemic control, however, this aim is not always achievable with brittle Type 1 diabetes. The focus on complications may also generate overwhelming concern about blindness, kidney failure or leg amputation, especially in those who are unable or unwilling to achieve blood glucose results within recommended levels. If this is the case, provision of information about the risk of complications is unhelpful as patients are already aware of the potential risk of prolonged hyperglycaemia. The provision of education and support that is specific to the individual's situation enables risk perception to be modified appropriately, accompanied by support for self-care behaviours. Scare tactics in diabetes health education are rarely successful.

'When I was shown pictures of diabetic foot ulcers by the diabetes nurse, it terrified me to the extent that I was scared to eat anything in case it put my blood sugar up. This just meant I had lots of hypos and developed nerve damage anyway – my consultant told me hypoglycaemia is more damaging than hyperglycaemia for the nerves, heart and brain'.

> 'My diabetologist used to lecture me about blindness and kidney failure all the time. It got to the stage where I dreaded going to clinic because of this, so I just stopped going to appointments. It was 17 years before I would go to another hospital diabetes clinic'.

Peripheral neuropathy and depression

Peripheral neuropathy is a chronic complication of diabetes, having two forms: diffuse neuropathy – commonly appearing as disorders of sensation in the extremities of the body; and distal polyneuropathy – affecting many nerves of the hands and feet. Frederick Pavy, a Victorian physician who studied the effects of diabetes, gave a well-observed description of the symptoms of peripheral neuropathy in the lower extremities of his patients with Type 2 diabetes, with no available treatment to reduce high blood glucose levels at that time (Pavy, 1885):

> "[Patients present with] Heavy legs, numb feet, lightning pain and deep-seated pain in the feet, extreme sensitivity to touch, muscle tenderness, and impairment of knee tendon reflexes."

We now recognise that those suffering nerve damage and neuropathic pain due to diabetes require psychological support as depression is common in these individuals (Vileikyte, et al., 2005). The relationship between the chronic pain of diabetic peripheral neuropathy and depression is clear, although other debilitating aspects of neuropathy which may induce depressive symptoms – such as unsteadiness on the feet and mobility limitations – have not been widely described (de Groot, et al., 2001). Unsurprisingly, depression is more common in those with a long-duration of diabetes and other comorbidities and/or complications associated with diabetes.

The degree of diabetic neuropathy cannot be seen by healthcare professionals and it is difficult to measure because pain is a subjective sensation. Many factors can affect the level of pain experienced, including the individual's pain tolerance, severity of neuropathy, presence of other health conditions, and personal coping mechanisms employed. Additionally, the presence of interleukin-6 increases the immune system inflammatory response in severe illness. This response is associated with the development of depressive symptoms – previously described as 'sickness behaviour' – where both pain and depression manifest (Danzer, 2001). The unpredictability of peripheral neuropathy pain and its varying duration is a major factor linked to depression associated with this condition (Vileikyte, et al., 2005).

Mood changes associated with glucose levels

As the primary energy source for the brain, a fine balance of glucose is necessary to avoid disruption to cerebral function. Glucose is toxic to the body in quantity and the brain struggles to function when glucose levels are too high or too low; this has a marked effect on mood, causing irritability, reducing wellbeing and cognitive dysfunction in people who have Type 1 or Type 2 diabetes. Sommerfield, et al. (2004) conducted research setting various tasks and using a questionnaire, demonstrating that short-term hyperglycaemia in Type 2 diabetes slows the speed of decision-making, impairing working memory and concentration, profoundly affecting mood status. This is also the case with acute hyperglycaemia and hypoglycaemia in Type 1 diabetes. For those with Type 2 diabetes and intermittent or chronic hyperglycaemia, an additional multiple risk of vascular disease – such as stroke – is present due to metabolic syndrome.

'My blood sugar is either too high or too low most of the time, rarely what it should be. Sometimes I have hyperglycaemia for days and for no particular reason, and it makes me very short-tempered with everything and everyone. I'm also slow to reply if asked something and I always have a terrible headache; doing even the simplest task is difficult, so I do it wrong. If I'm writing on the computer, my words are muddled and I make lots of spelling mistakes'.

'I'm Jekyll and Hyde with my Type 1. When I'm severely hypo or hyperglycaemic, I'm so nasty to the people I love and say really horrible things, flying into rages, screaming, stomping around, throwing things, and making a big deal about silly little things. One time, a tea-towel wasn't folded straight so that became a priority for me when my husband was telling me to test to see if I was having a hypo. Fortunately, he knows that isn't really me, but I absolutely hate myself afterwards and keep on apologising for being so horrible'.

'After 43 years of brittle Type 1 with many episodes of being unconscious, my short-term memory is terrible and I often mix words up – I laugh about it when it happens, but it does concern me because it's like having Alzheimer's, which my mother had'.

Research examining the effects of hyperglycaemia on the brain has reported confusion over words, reduced intelligence, altered mood state and impaired cognitive performance (Sommerfield, et al., 2004). Other studies show that hyperglycaemia reduces efficiency of brain networks (Dae-Jin, et al., 2016; McCrimmon, et al., 2012; Sporns, 2011). A further study involving individuals without diabetes demonstrated that a short-term high blood glucose reading of 17.8 mmol/L (320 dl/L) using an insulin clamp to prevent blood glucose reduction resulted in increased sensory nerve conduction and reduced motor nerve function (Sindrup, et al., 1988). High and low blood glucose levels therefore affect brain function in both diabetic and non-diabetic individuals.

Diabetes and other autoimmune diseases

Type 1 diabetes is an autoimmune condition where the immune system – which usually fights infection – attacks the insulin-producing cells of the pancreas and produces islet cell antibodies – proteins in the blood. These antibodies continue to destroy the insulin-producing beta cells for the rest of the individual's life with Type 1 diabetes because this auto-immune destruction is not reversible. However, onset of Type 1 diabetes can be temporarily delayed with treatments to reduce autoimmunity, but not indefinitely (Bluestone, et al., 2015). This immune system defect leads to the development of other autoimmune conditions – such as asthma, psoriasis, or hypothyroidism, known as polyautoimmunity; conversely, Type 1 diabetes tends to occur among individuals with pre-existing autoimmune conditions. The occurrence of further auto-immune diseases also increases with age due to the length of time the immune system has been dysfunctional (Cataldo and Marino, 2003).

The psychological consequences of coping with multiple health conditions has been under-reported as research tends to focus on self-management of only one condition, such as Type 1 diabetes following diagnosis. When subsequent chronic conditions are diagnosed, the individual is faced with adaptation to the further loss of health and the limitations this brings, learning to develop coping strategies if possible to help manage and deal with these increased and ongoing demands. In the case of Type 1 diabetes, the diabetes consultant will be familiar with polyautoimmunity, but when chronic conditions are both psychological and physical, there may be reduced understanding by healthcare professionals who have expertise in only one area of medicine.

Coeliac disease

Coeliac disease is a systemic condition that affects the whole body, not just the digestive tract. The condition is a chronic autoimmune disease triggered by an intolerance to gluten – a protein found in cereal grains such as wheat that is added to bread to make it rise. Gluten proteins are rich in glutamine and proline residues: proline proteins make gluten resistant to gastrointestinal digestion, creating an adverse inflammatory reaction in those with coeliac disease and gluten intolerance. In a study measuring the reaction to gluten proteins, individuals with coeliac disease were found to have an increased Coeliac Disease 4+ T-cell response to several distinct gluten peptides (Sollid, et al., 2012). Further research showed that individuals with coeliac disease produce specific antibodies making them intolerant to gluten proteins (Lauret and Rodrigo, 2013).

'I went to a pre-assessment appointment at a private hospital before having a keloid removed. I explained that I have Type I diabetes, coeliac disease, asthma, under-active thyroid, arthritis and depression. The lead nurse shook her head as if to say to her colleague, "This woman's going to be a problem". The assisting nurse kept apologising as she tried to take my blood. After five attempts, she called a doctor in to do it. The lead nurse then told me off for having poor veins and for taking up their time. She emphasised that the private hospital was a centre of excellence and that she was a senior nurse with "years of experience with people like me," adding that I should remember, "I was only the patient". I felt there was no professional competence and that I was being blamed – I just got a load of mental baggage from that appointment which comes back to me every time I have blood taken for annual HbA1c checks'.

Blood samples from those with coeliac disease characteristically show low levels of vitamin D due to intestinal malabsorption; this may also manifest as the autoimmune skin condition, psoriasis. Significantly increased polyautoimmunity has been seen in those with coeliac disease and their first-degree relatives when compared to individuals without the condition or a family history of the disease (Neuhausen, et al., 2008; Viljamada, et al., 2005; Catalado and Marino, 2003). Being diagnosed with coeliac disease early in life and having a family history of autoimmunity are risk factors for developing polyautoimmunity, while a gluten-free diet has been shown to have an anti-inflammatory effect on the small intestine (Cosnes, et al., 2008).

An increased prevalence of coeliac disease has been associated with other autoimmune disorders such as Type 1 diabetes, where 22 percent of individuals have both conditions or multiple autoimmune diseases (Triolo, et al., 2011; Stagi, et al., 2005). The development of poly-autoimmune conditions in addition to coeliac disease occurs because these diseases share a common pathogenic basis involving genetic sus-ceptibility and/or similar environmental triggers.

The association between coeliac disease and Type 1 diabetes mellitus has been studied extensively. These conditions are often seen together, or subsequently coeliac disease develops in those with Type 1 diabetes (Greco, et al., 2013; Cerutti, et al., 2004). Research suggests a pre-valence of coeliac disease among individuals with Type 1 diabetes of between 2.0–11 percent (Simsek, et al., 2013; Aggawal, et al., 2012). This risk is highest when Type 1 diabetes is diagnosed before four years of age. Prevalence of coeliac disease also increases with diabetes duration (Tiberti, et al., 2012; Pham-Short, et al., 2010). There is a second peak incidence of coeliac disease in those with Type 1 diabetes at age 45, so testing for the disease in adults is also necessary (Bakker, et al., 2013a). The diagnosis of coeliac disease as the primary condition is associated with an increased risk of developing secondary Type 1 diabetes in persons below the age of 20 (Ludvigsson, et al., 2006).

For younger individuals with both Type 1 diabetes and coeliac dis-ease, a gluten-free diet is recommended to prevent growth disorders due to malnutrition and to promote better glycaemic control by avoiding intestinal malabsorption (Camacara, et al., 2012; Abid, et al., 2011; Sponzilli, et al., 2010). However, gluten-free foods tend to be higher in carbohydrates so more insulin is required. Gluten has been found to trigger the development of vascular complications associated with dia-betes (Bakker, et al., 2013b; Leeds, et al., 2011). Poor nutrition, not maintaining a gluten-free diet, and immunoregulatory imbalance are associated with autoimmune conditions (Lauret and Rodrigo, 2013). Additionally, both Type 1 diabetes and coeliac disease exert a toll on bone metabolism, reducing bone density – osteopenia. Bone metabolism decreases with duration of diabetes and/or poor glycaemic control

(Lombardini, et al., 2010; Valerio, et al., 2008). The challenge of simultaneously managing Type 1 diabetes and coeliac disease is not always recognised by healthcare professionals.

Thyroid conditions

The thyroid gland lies close to the trachea in the throat and removes iodine – essential for cell metabolism – from the bloodstream in the form of iodide. Iodide combines with proteins in the thyroid gland to produce thyroxin and tri-iodothyronine. Both Type 1 diabetes and coeliac disease are increasingly common in those with autoimmune thyroid disease. Autoimmune thyroid conditions include hypothyroidism – an under-secretion of thyroid hormones by the thyroid gland due to autoimmune destruction; Graves' disease – an over-secretion of thyroid hormone due to enlargement of the thyroid gland; and Hashimoto's thyroiditis – where autoimmune attack causes under-secretion of thyroid hormone.

Prevalence of thyroid disorders in those with existing autoimmune conditions ranges from 2.0–25 percent (Spadaccino, et al., 2008; Hadithi, et al., 2007; Ch'ng, et al., 2007). Thyroid disease is diagnosed in a quarter of individuals with coeliac disease and/or Type 1 diabetes; and the risk of developing thyroid disease is three times more likely because of an existing autoimmune disorder when compared to those without autoimmune disease (Meloni, et al., 2009; Elfstrom, et al., 2008; Ch'ng, et al., 2007).

'I've had several really bad hospital experiences for operations where having Type 1 diabetes, coeliac disease and an under-active thyroid just seemed to completely throw the surgical staff. One time, they didn't order me a gluten-free diabetic diet, so my husband had to bring food in. They also took away my insulin pens and thyroxin, giving me insulin when they felt it was necessary – which completely upset my glycaemic control. Because I was feeling terrible after the surgery, I didn't have the strength to argue. There was no speedy assistance when I told a nurse I was having a bad hypo, so I ate some sugar from sachets my husband had tucked into my dressing gown pocket for emergencies. That hospital stay made me so stressed and anxious because I handed over my care to people who seemed to know nothing about my conditions'.

Excessive thyroid hormones impact on glucose metabolism, causing hyperglycaemia. Hyperthyroidism – over-production of thyroid hormones, has a detrimental effect on insulin, reducing its working time and effectiveness. Individuals with diabetes and hyperthyroidism require more insulin to prevent hyperglycaemia if excess thyroxin levels are not controlled. Untreated hyperthyroidism is associated with a reduced level of C-peptide – an inactive building block of insulin – to pro-insulin ratio, suggesting an association between excess thyroxin and abnormal processing of pro-insulin in those with an over-active thyroid condition (Beer, et al., 1989). The association between hyperglycaemia and the over-production of thyroid hormones is due to the increase in glucose absorption in the gut.

The production of glucose by the body in those with and without diabetes is enhanced in a number of ways when the individual has hyperthyroidism. An excess of thyroid hormones causes an increase in the concentration of glucose in the liver, raising its glucose output, leading to abnormal glucose metabolism (Hage, et al., 2011). In addition, an increase in protein synthesis and the mobilisation of fat – lipolysis – is associated with increased levels of thyroid hormones. In turn, gluconeogenesis occurs – the generation of glucose from non-carbohydrate sources by the liver. Hyperthyroidism is known to increase levels of glucagon, making the liver release stored glucose quickly; growth hormone and catecholamine levels – substances that raise blood glucose levels in response to stress, further contributing to impaired glucose tolerance.

If one hormone level is disrupted, this causes an increase or decrease in other hormones. A fine balance exists between levels of insulin and thyroid hormones: if thyroxin is over- or under-produced, blood glucose levels are affected because carbohydrate metabolism is compromised. Individuals with Type 1 diabetes may also suffer from hypothyroid or hyperthyroid conditions due to autoimmune abnormality. The existence of hyperthyroidism associated thyrotoxicosis – overproduction of thyroid hormones – and Type 1 diabetes leads to poor glycaemic control, with increased episodes of diabetic ketoacidosis due to hyperglycaemia (Sola, et al., 2002).

Hyperthyroidism impacts heavily on the individual's mental health, their ability to stay focused and relate well with others. Serious mental health issues, academic failure, and dangerous risk-taking behaviors and lapses in judgment can be the presenting signs of an overactive thyroid. It's important that parents and healthcare professionals consider this when evaluating a child, teenager or adult with these problems (Ponder, 2017).

The under-production of thyroid hormones in hypothyroidism also affects blood glucose levels. The liver produces less glucose in those with Type 1 diabetes and hypothyroidism, meaning that less insulin is required. However, when thyroid function is normalised with medication, this may lead to higher blood glucose levels and adverse effects on glycemic control if insulin dosages are not increased accordingly.

Individuals with Type 1 diabetes may experience frequent and unexplained hypoglycaemia due to hypothyroidism; this is reversed with the commencement of thyroxin medication. However, some studies show that hypothyroidism has no effect on the activity of insulin (Maratou, et al., 2009; Dimitriardis, et al., 2006; Cettour-Rose, et al., 2005). Frequent hypoglycaemia and associated hypothyroidism is thought to be due to the way body tissues use glucose rather than a reduction in thyroid hormones (Lai, et al., 2011).

Undiagnosed hypothyroidism can also cause dramatic swings in blood glucose levels between hypo- and hyperglycaemia in brittle Type 1 diabetes. A causal link has been identified between increased levels of thyroid stimulating hormone – TSH – resulting in hypothyroidism, and the development of metabolic syndrome – biochemical and physical abnormalities normally associated with the development of cardiovascular disease and Type 2 diabetes (Erdogan, et al., 2011; Lai, et al., 2011).

'I was diagnosed with an under-active thyroid after having Type 1 diabetes for 25 years. I'd been very tired, had no energy for a long time and my brain seemed very slow. With low-dose thyroxin and blood tests every three months, I didn't feel any different and I was told that the condition was getting worse. My diabetes consultant said I wasn't looking after myself properly and warned that my mild sight problems would become serious. I researched low thyroid levels, mentioning to my GP that it could cause high blood sugars. He adamantly disagreed that my thyroid was the problem, which was very frustrating. An endocrinologist agreed with me in the end'.

An under-active thyroid gland has been shown to increase the risk of neuropathy in those with Type 2 diabetes (Chen, et al., 2007). Contrary to the understanding that high levels of thyroid hormone are associated with hyperglycaemia, this finding assumes an increase in blood glucose levels in association with low levels of thyroid hormone, triggering diabetes complications. Neuropathy may occur because Type 2 diabetes develops as a result of metabolic syndrome and adverse changes to the metabolism – controlled by thyroid hormones, potentially explaining hyperglycaemia.

> 'I developed sight problems associated with my Type 1 diabetes and Graves' disease, with awful headaches and eye pain. This meant I was forced to give up my job as a driving instructor. My whole life and body had fallen apart. After about a year during which I became very depressed – affecting my blood glucose levels – I began intravenous steroid treatment. Eventually, the headaches and eye pain went, but I had to re-train for another career. I still resent the life changes ill-health has burdened me with and I'm still taking depression medication'.

There may also be a connection with unsynchronised insulin and thyroid hormone levels in Type 2 diabetes, although this is not an autoimmune condition like Type 1. For individuals with diabetic nephropathy, renal function when taking thyroxin has been found to improve (Den Hollander, et al., 2005; Singer, et al., 2001), although diabetic retinopathy appeared to worsen with the condition (Yang, et al., 2010). It is also the case that when the blood vessels of the eyes are compromised in diabetes, this makes the optic nerve more susceptible to pressure exerted by the enlargement of the extraocular muscles – a condition known as dysthyroid optic neuropathy, due to changes to the eye in Graves' disease (Kamboj, et al., 2017). This can be distressing for the individual.

There is a clear association between autoimmune thyroid conditions and Type 1 diabetes: this relationship has adverse implications in respect of impaired growth and development in young individuals, with adverse effects on growth and cell metabolism. As with other chronic health conditions, early detection of both Type 1 diabetes and autoimmune thyroid disorders enables treatment and maintenance of the disease to delay or reduce the impact of further physical and mental health problems.

Addison's disease

An adrenal gland is situated on top of each kidney. The kidneys' outer layers secrete a number of hormones: mineralcorticoids such as aldosterone which increase the uptake of sodium and the secretion of potassium; glucocorticoids – such as hydrocortisone – known as cortisol, and androgens – sex hormones. Addison's disease – also known as chronic cortical hypofunction or adrenocortical insufficiency – develops due to gradual autoimmune destruction of the adrenal cortex. Addison's disease can take many years to develop and may only be obvious in the middle-aged with the development of increased skin pigmentation due to a lack of corticosteroids.

Other indicators include a greater amount of sodium being lost in the urine with an associated rise in levels of blood potassium; and hypoglycaemia. The latter is most frequently associated with Type 1 diabetes when there is an excess of blood insulin. However, individuals with Type 2 diabetes may also develop hypoglycaemia if blood glucose lowering medication is taken without food or if prolonged physical exercise has been undertaken, reducing blood glucose levels further. Treatment of Addison's disease is by replacement of corticosteroids in the form of hydrocortisone, which may be required for a long duration. There is also a more severe form of Addison's disease, a medical emergency known as acute adrenocortical hypofunction – also called Addisonian crisis or adrenal crisis. This occurs due to a rapid reduction in hydrocortisone if the individual has an infection or when steroid therapy is omitted. The individual loses consciousness, requiring rapid intravenous infusion of hydrocortisone (UCLA, 2020).

In 2018, 8,400 UK individuals had Addison's disease; it is most common between the ages of 30 and 50 and more so in women than men (NHS, 2018). However, the condition is five times more common in those with Type 1 diabetes as a concomitant autoimmune condition, and 10–18 percent of those with Type 1 diabetes will also develop Addison's (McAuley and Frier, 1999). However, the occurrence of Type 1 diabetes in those with Addison's disease is much lower at only 1.2 percent (Schneider, 2019). Type 1 diabetes therefore precedes the development of adrenocortical insufficiency in the majority of cases.

McAuley and Frier (1999) reported the case of a 19-year old man with Type 1 diabetes and autoimmune hypothyroidism. He began to experience disabling and frequent low blood glucose levels over several months, despite reducing his insulin dosage considerably. His recurrent hypoglycaemia was found to be due to adrenal insufficiency decreasing hormones such as cortisol which maintains the levels of glucose in blood plasma. This case study shows that undiagnosed Addison's disease can cause severe hypoglycaemia due to its influence on glycaemic control.

If there is an overall reduction in insulin requirement by 15–20 percent corresponding with continual low glucose readings, underlying Addison's disease is indicated. The individual also has abnormal skin pigmentation and – in young and adolescent patients – a lack of growth, meaning that investigation of these symptoms should also involve thyroid function tests as polyautoimmunity often exists with Addison's disease, thyroid dysfunction and Type 1 diabetes.

Individuals with Addison's disease are also at risk of developing coeliac disease (Myhre, et al., 2013; O'Leary, et al., 2002). Research shows a 5.0–12 percent prevalence of coeliac disease in those with pre-existing Addison's disease (Myhre, et al., 2013; Betterle, et al., 2006; Biagi, et al., 2006). Conversely, there is also an increased risk of Addison's disease among those with coeliac disease (Elfstrom, et al., 2007). Although vital in managing coeliac disease, adopting a gluten-free diet does not alter the natural history of Addison's disease (Betterle, et al., 2006), therefore this does not offer any protection from the onset of this secondary auto-immune condition.

There is an uncommon endocrine disorder known as Schmidt's syndrome – or autoimmune polyglandurar syndrome Type 2 – describing Addison's disease with autoimmune thyroid disease and/or Type 1 diabetes mellitus; Schmidt's syndrome has an estimated prevalence of 1.4 percent (Betterle, et al., 2002). Symptoms in those with this cluster of conditions have been misdiagnosed as a generalised anxiety and depression once Type 1 diabetes, Addison's disease and thyroiditis become stabilised with treatment (Betterle, et al., 1996). The syndrome usually affects women in their forties after several years of poly-autoimmunity. Symptoms of this disorder comprise difficulty concentrating, insomnia and progressively worsening intermittent fatigue. Prompt diagnosis and treatment can prevent serious complications and improve quality of life.

Asthma

Asthma is characterised by breathlessness when there is generalised narrowing of the airways throughout the lungs. In terms of the cause, asthma may be extrinisic, where external allergens, such as pollen, dust or smoke trigger an attack, or intrinsic, where there is no apparent external cause. Asthma can be:

- Episodic – where attacks occur at any time, of variable length and severity.
- Chronic – where the individual has persistent wheezing, coughing and permanent breathlessness with frequent chest infections.
- Status asthmaticus – where the attack is severe and lasts longer than 24 hours with no response to medication, leading to an increased heart rate and potential loss of conciseness.

There is undoubtedly a negative association between Type 1 diabetes and asthma symptoms. Developed countries have an increased prevalence of concomitant Type 1 diabetes and asthma (Hsia, et al., 2015) and an upsurge in autoimmune diseases as a whole (Benchimol, et al., 2015). This could be explained by the nature of these chronic health conditions and their treatments. Complex immune response interactions play a role in the development of both asthma and Type 1 diabetes (Hsia, et al., 2015), which occurs due to viral infection. The immune response is altered, attacking both the infection and the insulin-producing beta cells, responding adversely to triggers such as house dust in the case of asthma. Individuals with both conditions exhibit lower levels of immune system components so that it works less efficiently (Marianna, et al., 2006).

A significantly higher number of cases of asthma have been seen in those with Type 1 diabetes than in the general population. The risk of developing asthma is highest in children under eight years of age, and those hospitalised for Type 1 diabetes emergencies more than twice per year are more likely to develop asthma (Yung-Tshung, et al., 2015). Individuals with Type 1 diabetes and fewer than two hospitalisations per year are not at increased risk. This implies that the immune system is adversely affected by the extreme metabolic upset that is ketoacidosis, requiring emergency treatment to reverse the altered pH balance associated with prolonged hyperglycaemia during infection, or deliberate and frequent insulin omissions.

It is known that the asthma treatment, Salbutamol – also known as Ventolin – stimulates the pancreas to produce more insulin; this may be a factor in the later development of Type 1 diabetes. Poorer pulmonary function among individuals with diabetes has been noted when compared to those without diabetes (Walter, et al., 2003). Individuals with Type 1 diabetes who subsequently develop asthma may do so due to a reduced exposure to immune-system strengthening factors at a younger age – a theory termed the 'hygiene hypothesis'. Poor glycaemic control is also a contributory factor, increasing susceptibility to ongoing autoimmune disease by impairing an already dysfunctional immune system as high blood glucose levels increase chronic inflammation, disrupting regulatory T-cell responses. Both Type 1 diabetes and asthma share the same risk factors, while a low childhood bodyweight has also been suggested as a reason why children with Type 1 diabetes go on to develop asthma, it is also the case that young persons with both conditions tend to have higher HbA1c levels than those with Type 1 diabetes alone (Black, et al., 2011).

Concurrent asthma and diabetes self-management decisions may be influenced by psychological factors such as health beliefs, attitudes, or emotions, as well as the presence of any co-occurring mental health conditions. As we have previously seen, depression is associated with decreased problem-solving ability, reduced capability to perform complex tasks, and poor memory and attention span. Decisions made during attacks of slow-onset asthma are impaired, even with theoretical knowledge of appropriate action (Lehrer, et al., 2002). Anxiety can also adversely affect asthma and diabetes by influencing self-management behaviour, impairing the autonomic and immune systems. In contrast, low levels of disease-specific anxiety may lead to increased asthma and/ or diabetes morbidity as the individual's anxiety may be needed to motivate prompt treatment initiation.

Arthritis

Due to wear and tear on the bones and joints, osteoarthritis is very common, especially in weight-bearing knee and hip joints or following trauma, e.g., a broken wrist. Extra bone then forms to compensate for this degeneration which narrows the spaces between the joints, with cysts forming under the bone surface. The condition is treated with anti-inflammatory medication and physiotherapy to manage joint stiffness.

The nature of diabetes affects bone metabolism, changing the structure of the skeleton more frequently than in the non-diabetic population. In the same way, diabetes may affect the musculo-skeletal system: the breakdown of proteins into glucose – glycosylation – occurs due to abnormal blood glucose levels, causing an accumulation of strengthening collagen which changes the structure of connective tissues (Kim, et al., 2001). This is most frequently seen among individuals with long-duration Type 1 diabetes, although there is an association between increased collagen and Type 2 diabetes where there is more stress on weight-bearing joints due to obesity.

Autoimmune arthritic changes associated with diabetes – known as cheiroarthopathy – often affect the small joints of the hands, causing stiffening and reduced mobility due to over-production of collagen and joint degeneration. This complication is seen in 50 percent of individuals with Type 1 diabetes (Arkkila, et al., 1994) and Type 2 patients (Arkkila, et al., 1997). The condition is strongly associated with an increased risk of developing proliferative retinopathy and neuropathy in those with either Type 1 or Type 2 diabetes. Individuals with Type 2 and cheiroarthopathy also have a greater risk of macrovascular disease and poor glycaemic control.

Stiffening of the joints in the fingers is exclusively seen in diabetes and can occur soon after the diagnosis of Type 1 in young individuals as well as in those with a long duration of the disease (Clarke, et al., 1990). This outcome can be extremely debilitating, severely affecting quality of life due to the imposed limitations. Treatment in such cases consists of corticosteroid injections and surgery to reduce the overgrowth of collagen in these joints (Aljanlan, et al., 1999). Individuals with diabetes are especially prone to a form of arthritis known as calcific periarthritis where deposits of calcium appear in the soft tissues around the shoulders (Lehmer and Ragsdale, 2012).

Due to weight-bearing, arthritic changes are frequently observed in the feet of individuals with diabetes, such as diabetic osteoarthropathy and Charcot neuropathic arthropathy. There is a causal link between Type 2 diabetes, obesity and osteoarthritis in the weight-bearing bones of the feet (Kim, et al., 2001). Neuropathic arthropathy – also known as Charcot joints – describes the degeneration of any joint, but the condition most commonly occurs in the lower extremity at the foot and ankle (Shah, 2020). These arthritic changes affect the individual's gait and change the shape of the foot causing mobility and footwear problems, having an adverse impact on quality of life – as shown in the comment below.

'One morning when I woke, my left foot had swollen to twice the size of the right. My doctor had no advice other than to rest it, which was impossible as I had a busy job on my feet all day and children to care for at home. I bought a pair of roomy boots and there was no pain when I walked – the swelling lasted for a year. I was left with arthritic claw toes, a dislocated big toe and a huge pressure point on the sole of my foot. It's now very painful to walk as my toes crack and the changes are permanent. I now know this is due to my poorly managed diabetes, and find it very depressing and difficult to accept – my GP should have urgently referred me to someone before it got this bad. He never even asked about my blood glucose control'.

Psoriasis

Psoriasis is an autoimmune condition affecting the skin and joints. This presents as red, flaky, crusty patches covered with silvery scales on the elbows, knees, scalp and lower back that are often itchy, accompanied by joint degeneration. Although Type 2 diabetes is not an autoimmune condition, psoriasis is associated with an increase in the production of insulin to reduce blood glucose levels and the subsequent development of Type 2 diabetes (Fitzgerald, et al., 2014). Research shows that obesity – defined as a body mass index of 30> – increases the risk of developing moderate to severe psoriasis (Bremmer, et al., 2010; Sterry, et al., 2007).

Psoriasis has also been linked to metabolic syndrome: a group of physical states and cardiovascular risk factors including abdominal obesity; impaired glucose regulation; high levels of triglyceride blood fats; reduced high-density lipid blood fats; and high blood pressure (Jensen, et al., 2013; Tam, et al., 2008; Cohen, et al., 2007).

Comorbid Type 1 or Type 2 diabetes and psoriasis increases the individual's risk of experiencing earlier onset cardiovascular events (Boencke, et al., 2011; Mehta, et al., 2010; Tobin, et al., 2010; Neimann, et al., 2006). Additionally, growing evidence shows that psoriasis is more likely to develop when the individual has insulin resistance (Brauchli, et al., 2008).

Insulin resistance is defined as the phenomenon where there is reduced glucose absorption by cells stimulated by insulin (Boencke, el al., 2011). Blood glucose levels then rise, signaling the production of more insulin, although there are already abnormally high insulin levels present which cannot be utilised. The insulin-producing cells of the pancreas become over-worked and eventually fail, at which point Type 2 diabetes develops. Decreased sensitivity to insulin in cases of psoriasis leads to vasoconstriction of the arteries and earlier artery disease (Balchi, et al., 2010; Karadag, et al., 2010).

In obese individuals with psoriasis and insulin resistance, fat tissue macrophages – cells that remove bacteria and foreign bodies from blood and tissues – can also significantly destabilise glucose metabolism to contribute to the development of Type 2 diabetes. Substances called resistin, adiponectin, adipokines and leptin are also present in abnormal quantities in association with obesity. Resistin is released by the fat cells to fight the action of insulin on the cells, preventing the lowering of blood glucose. Levels of resistin are raised in psoriasis and diminished with phototherapy, a treatment commonly used to improve the condition (Boehncke, et al., 2012). High resistin levels increase the likelihood of insulin resistance and Type 2 diabetes as there is more fat tissue with obesity. Leptin is a hormone made by fat cells that works to regulate body fat. Leptin deficiency is a pathological cause of obesity, although when the obesity is due to excess food consumption and a sedentary lifestyle, leptin levels are increased, and this becomes a risk factor for Type 2 diabetes (Klok, et al., 2007). Individuals with psoriasis have higher leptin levels when compared to those without the condition (Chen, et al., 2008; Johnston, et al., 2008; Wang, et al., 2008).

Adiponectin is a hormone produced by the fat cells that causes the tissues to be sensitive to insulin. It has both anti-inflammatory and anti-atherogenic effects – reducing fatty deposits in the arteries (Takahashi, et al., 2008). Those with both Type 2 diabetes and psoriasis have lower adiponectin levels (Fitzgerald, et al., 2014), although no connection has been made regarding the causality or severity of either chronic health condition (Shibata, et al., 2009; Takahashi, et al., 2008). Adipokines are known to cause Type 2 diabetes, high blood pressure and narrowing of the arteries. While there is a clear association between the adipokines produced by excess fat tissue and insulin resistance in Type 2 diabetes, the link between psoriasis and diabetes independent of obesity is not explained by the presence of adipokines.

Inflammation associated with psoriasis may not only impair insulin, but also contribute to the development of insulin resistance (Fitzgerald, et al., 2014), the development of atherosclerotic plaque in the arteries and ongoing inflammation. Atherosclerosis – narrowing – due to plaque formation is also a chronic complication of diabetes, eventually leading to coronary heart disease. A further inflammatory antagonist is interleukin-6 which is also associated with glucose intolerance (Eder, et al., 2009), levels being raised when there is coexisting obesity and psoriasis and increasing further as psoriasis worsens (Coimbra, et al., 2010). The medications, Exenatide and Liraglutide used to treat Type 2 diabetes have been found to reduce itching, inflammation and insulin resistance in cases of psoriasis. This is possibly because excess glucose is a toxin in the body, causing irritation and itching.

Psychological aspects of psoriasis

Because the appearance of psoriasis on the skin may be difficult to conceal, it can be a very distressing autoimmune condition, resulting in psychological consequences. Research shows that 37–88 percent of individuals agree their psoriasis is caused or worsened by stress (Fortune, et al., 1998; Al'Abadie, et al., 1994). Life stresses lead to worsening of psoriasis with increased itching, while excessive worry increases susceptibility to the effects of stress (Verhoeven, et al., 2009b; Fortune, et al., 2003). The hormonal response to stress involves an increase in histamine levels and inflammatory substances by the immune system, triggering 'sickness behaviour' and depressive symptoms.

The term, 'sickness behaviour' describes a coordinated set of behaviour changes that develop in all cases of illness, including low motivation to eat, listlessness, fatigue, malaise, a reduced interest in social activity, altered sleep patterns, inability to experience pleasure, an exaggerated response to pain and poor concentration (Dantzer, 2004; 2001). These behaviours are the same as those experienced during depression, although there is a reason for this if triggered by illness. Conversely, a diagnosis of clinical depression is based on there being no discernible reason for symptoms, such as illness or bereavement.

Depression is experienced by over one-third of those with psoriasis (Weiss, et al., 2002; Fortune, et al., 2000). Gupta, et al., (1993) reported suicidal thoughts in 5.5 percent of individuals with the condition, while 9.5 percent expressed their wish to die – psoriasis steroid medication can cause psychological imbalance. A large UK study showed increased diagnoses of depression, anxiety and suicidality when compared to individuals without psoriasis; this study estimated that over 10,400 diagnoses of depression; 7,100 diagnoses of anxiety, and 350 diagnoses of suicidality are attributable to psoriasis each year (Kurd, et al., 2010).

The individual's psoriasis health beliefs have been cited as the cause of psychological distress. Mizra, et al. (2012) suggest those with psoriasis are likely to feel vulnerability to harm, defectiveness, social isolation-predicted anxiety and depression. Although there is strong evidence associating depression and anxiety with psoriasis, much of the guidance regarding diagnosis and management – as with diabetes – fails to include routine screening for anxiety and depression, meaning that the individual may not receive the support they need.

Treatment for those with psoriasis and depressive symptoms involves a medication – TNF-a antagonists – used to suppress the immune system response causing inflammation of the skin. The amount of medication is raised during a period of depression (Himmerich, et al., 2008) and this has been linked to feeling tired, potentially explaining the association between depression and fatigue (Illman, et al., 2005). TNF-a antagonists are both safe and favourable in improving physical and psychological symptoms of psoriasis (Revicki, et al., 2008; Shikar, et al., 2007; Gordon, et al., 2006). However, this treatment does not reverse depressive symptoms in those with psoriasis (Kimball, et al., 2012; Himmerich, et al., 2008).

Individuals with psoriasis treated with anti-depressant and corticosteroid medication show improvement in their physical and psychological symptoms compared with corticosteroid use alone (Alpsoy, et al., 1998). This is not the case for the anti-depressant, Fluoxetine, suitable for the treatment of depression in those with diabetes but exacerbating symptoms of psoriasis (Tan, et al, 2010; Tamer, et al, 2009; Hemlock, et al, 1992). This can also be said of Bupropion (Cox, et al, 2002) and Lithium (Basayari, et al, 2010).

'When my psoriasis was very bad I was admitted to hospital. I totally withdrew from society and was told by a psychologist that some people use long-term illness as a place they can retreat into to avoid the world. This was true – I didn't know I was doing this: I didn't leave the house when my face was covered with peeling, scabby patches because people would stare. I stopped seeing friends and handed in my notice at work – my joints hurt and I couldn't move easily. With strong psoriasis medication and CBT, my symptoms improved enough for me to leave hospital after ten weeks. I had to force myself to go to the shops rather than have home deliveries and contacted friends again, although one turned her back on me, saying I'd shut her out and ignored her'.

Few interventions have targeted the effect of stress on psoriasis, or the impact of stress on the immune system. Psychological interventions may address cognitive and behavioural processes: cognitive behaviour therapy, or stress reduction – arousal reduction. Meta-analysis of eight psychological interventions for individuals with skin conditions found that the studies were small and poorly designed (Lavda, et al., 2012). Interventions with differing aims had little effect on the individual and outcomes could not be compared with one another.

Diabetes comorbidities

A comorbidity describes a physical or mental disease or condition that coexists with a primary disease. Comorbid conditions can contribute to overall health and wellbeing, having an impact on treatment; any comorbid condition can greatly complicate the disease. In association with Type 2 diabetes, comorbidities such as obesity, hypertension, liver disease and sleep apnoea are common. Iglay, et al., (2016) found that 98 percent of 1.3 million adults with Type 2 diabetes had at least one comorbid chronic condition and almost 90 percent had at least two – multimorbidities. Certain diseases can increase the risk of developing diabetes while conversely, diabetes can sometimes develop before a comorbid condition. Several conditions are closely associated with Type 2 diabetes:

Hypertension

The global prevalence of hypertension is high, and treatment of hypertension is the most common use of chronic prescription medications (Muntner, et al., 2018). Hypertension is a condition where blood pressure regularly measures above 130 mmHg systolic and 80 mmHg diastolic. High blood pressure is an extremely common comorbidity of diabetes, being dependent on obesity, ethnicity and age; De Boer, et al. (2017) found that up to three-quarters of people with diabetes also have hypertension. The two conditions share many of the same risk factors, such as obesity and having a sedentary lifestyle; high blood pressure is also associated with insulin resistance, which can be described as a state of pre-diabetes, this condition being a precursor to Type 2 diabetes.

In patients assigned to lower blood pressure targets of 80 mmHg, improved outcomes were achieved, especially in preventing stroke (UKPDS Group, 1998; Kjeldsen, et al., 1998), demonstrating the benefit of targeting a diastolic blood pressure of ≤80 mmHg. It is clear that blood pressure readings ≥120/70 mmHg are associated with increased cardiovascular events and mortality in those with diabetes. Risk continues to decrease to within the normal range with a target blood pressure of <130/80 mmHg, if it can be safely achieved; achieving lower levels, however, increases the potential for medication side-effects and the cost of care (American Diabetes Association, 2003).

Obesity

Comorbidities are not necessarily symptoms of the primary condition, but may still be very closely related to it. Obesity is defined as an abnormal or excessive accumulation of body fat that negatively affects health; this may be a causal factor or may occur in conjunction with diabetes. Obesity is believed to be a promoter of Type 2 diabetes mellitus. Malone and Hansen (2019) recently found that obesity is not the cause of Type 2 diabetes as insulin resistance can occur in the muscle of lean individuals not predisposed to diabetes before they become obese; this insulin resistance is the cause of excessive fat accumulation, not because of it. Malone and Hansen (2019) confirm that this early muscle insulin resistance is also responsible for hyperlipidaemia and excess fat accumulation seen in Type 2 diabetes.

Dyslipidaemia

Dyslipidemia describes abnormal levels of the high-density lipoproteins (HDL) that function to help remove low-density lipoproteins (LDL) from the blood; this may be genetic and/or related to lifestyle factors. Dyslipidemia shares many of the same risk factors as diabetes and is an extremely common comorbidity (Schofield, et al., 2016). Dyslipidemia is divided into primary and secondary types: primary dyslipidemia is inherited, while secondary dyslipidemia is an acquired condition developing from other causes, such as obesity or Type 2 diabetes.

Mixed hyperlipidaemia

Mixed hyperlipidaemia describes genetically elevated levels of cholesterol, triglycerides, and other blood fats, raising the risk of coronary heart disease, peripheral vascular disease, stroke, and premature heart attacks. Mixed hyperlipidaemia is often associated with metabolic syndrome, non-alcoholic fatty liver disease, and risk of developing Type 2 diabetes. This condition affects 1–2 percent of the population and is the most commonly inherited lipid disorder; mixed hyperlipidaemia is exacerbated by diabetes, hypothyroidism, obesity, and alcohol abuse. Blood tests indicate lower-than-average HDL cholesterol levels and higher levels of LDL cholesterol, triglycerides, and apolipoprotein B100 (Viljoen, 2011). The treatment goal is to reduce the risk of heart disease and its complications; the treatment plan is dependent on age at diagnosis, lipid levels and the presence of symptoms, such as chest pain.

Lifestyle changes alone can help reduce cholesterol and triglyceride levels.

Non-alcoholic fatty liver disease (NAFLD)

NAFLD is marked by elevated liver enzymes and enlargement of the organ due to an accumulation of fat; risk of NAFLD increases with obesity and abdominal fat and may develop as a comorbidity of Type 2 diabetes (Dharmalingam and Yamasandhi, 2018). If left untreated, NAFLD can cause scarring, an increased risk of liver failure, and liver cancer. Type 2 diabetes mellitus and non-alcoholic fatty liver disease are common comorbidities; NAFLD has been regarded as a manifestation of metabolic syndrome. Presentations of NAFLD range from simple steatosis, non-alcoholic steatohepatitis (NASH), and cirrhosis. NAFLD has a 70 percent prevalence among Type 2 diabetes patients (Dharmalingam and Yamasandhi, 2018).

Overweight/obesity and insulin resistance have been strongly associated with NAFLD. Age, sex, liver function test, platelet count, lipid profile, BMI, and ultrasound/MRI, are useful in the early detection and staging of NAFLD, and predicting fibrosis. Many of the same lifestyle measures that help manage Type 2 diabetes can also help to reverse non-alcoholic fatty liver disease, including improving insulin resistance with good glycaemic control by following a healthy diet, increasing physical activity, and weight loss.

Obstructive sleep apnoea

Obstructive sleep apnoea (OSA) is a common disorder describing repeated complete or partial upper airway obstructions during sleep and continual cessation of breathing, leading to reduced blood oxygen levels. This condition may be caused by a partial collapse of the airway due to excess weight or obesity. Diabetes is considered a risk factor for sleep apnoea, but it may also be a comorbidity (American Diabetes Association, 2020). Multiple studies have indicated that OSA may be a risk factor for the development of Type 2 diabetes independent of obesity and other confounders: interruptions to sleep are a key part of Type 2 diabetes risk (Subramanian, et al., 2019). The relationship between OSA and Type 2 diabetes is two-way: Studies have shown that Type 2 diabetes might lead to the development of OSA as a result of the effect of insulin resistance and autonomic dysfunction on upper airways stability (Horner, 2012; Balkau, et al., 2010).

Treatment to manage the signs and symptoms of OSA include behavioral approaches to improving sleep habits and weight control; both medical and surgical weight loss significantly reduce the severity of OSA. More recently, weight loss related to lifestyle interventions in those with Type 2 diabetes has been shown to significantly improve OSA severity (Kuna, et al., 2013).

Preventing comorbidities in diabetes

The risk of developing comorbidities of Type 2 diabetes can be significantly reduced by modifying the lifestyle factors that increase risk, such as:

- Maintaining a healthy weight (and losing weight if necessary)
- Smoking cessation
- Being physically active
- Good glycaemic control
- Getting adequate sleep
- Reducing stress

Regular screening for pre-diabetes can identify conditions earlier in their development, helping to prevent full-blown diseases.

Managing comorbidities in diabetes

Having multiple comorbidities means that the individual must visit additional healthcare professionals for those conditions, and this care may be coordinated by the diabetes specialist. It is necessary that all healthcare providers be up-to-date with current medications, bloodwork, and treatment schedules (Algoblan, et al., 2014). Lifestyle changes can help prevent comorbid conditions from developing alongside diabetes as well as treating them. It's never too late for the individual to make lifestyle changes to better manage blood glucose levels.

Key messages in this chapter:

- Type 1 diabetes is an autoimmune condition where the immune system attacks the insulin-producing cells of the pancreas and produces islet cell antibodies.
- Increased prevalence of coeliac disease has been associated with other autoimmune disorders, such as Type 1 diabetes. The development of polyautoimmune conditions occurs because these

diseases share a common pathogenic basis involving genetic susceptibility and/or similar environmental triggers.

- Thyroid disease is diagnosed in a quarter of individuals with coeliac disease and/or Type 1 diabetes; the risk of developing thyroid disease is three times more likely in those with existing autoimmune disorder.
- Addison's disease can take many years to develop and may only be obvious in the middle-aged with the development of increased skin pigmentation, due to a lack of corticosteroids.
- A significantly higher number of cases of asthma have been seen in those with Type 1 diabetes than in the general population.
- Reduced joint mobility due to over-production of collagen is seen in 50 percent of individuals with either Type 1 or Type 2 diabetes; this is strongly associated with developing proliferative retinopathy and neuropathy.
- Inflammation associated with psoriasis may not only impair the action of insulin, but also contribute to the development of insulin resistance.
- Sickness behaviour describes a coordinated set of behaviour changes that develop in all cases of illness, including low motivation to eat, listlessness, fatigue, malaise, a reduced interest in social activity, altered sleep patterns, inability to experience pleasure, an exaggerated response to pain and poor concentration.
- Chronic complications frequently occur in those with long-duration diabetes due to altered metabolic parameters, and complications can still develop in those with well-controlled diabetes.
- Having multiple comorbidities means the individual must visit additional healthcare professionals for those conditions; this care may be coordinated by the diabetes specialist. It is necessary that all healthcare providers be up-to-date with current medications, bloodwork, and treatment schedules.

7   Diabetes, Stigma and Weight Loss Surgery

Type 2 diabetes accounts for 90 percent of diagnoses of diabetes worldwide. The current rise in cases of Type 2 diabetes is fuelled by physical inactivity and obesity as these are the primary risk factors for developing metabolic syndrome – insulin resistance, high blood pressure, overweight or obesity and high levels of blood fats. For the individual, there is stigma – recognising others as different – where Type 2 is regarded by society as 'self-induced'. Similar to perceived self-blame following the diagnosis of diabetic complications, some with Type 2 diabetes have been stigmatised by health professionals and misunderstood by those with Type 1 diabetes whose condition has an autoimmune cause rather than as a result of obesity and lifestyle choice. This is demonstrated in the following comments from people with Type 2 diabetes.

Victim blaming

> 'At diabetes clinic one time a man got aggressive with me, shouting that there was nothing he could do about his Type 1 diabetes, while if I lost some weight, I could get rid of my Type 2'.
>
> 'I've been told several times by nurses, doctors and dieticians that it's in my own hands, that I've given myself Type 2 diabetes because I'm lacking self-control, motivation to exercise, and that I obviously don't care about my body and what I eat'.

This victim-blaming attitude that some people with Type 2 diabetes experience suggests there is potential to change eating and exercise

DOI: 10.4324/9781003260219-8

behaviour in order to reverse the life-threatening consequences of Type 2 diabetes – such as heart disease. Individuals with Type 2 diabetes may fail to understand their condition and its associated risks, despite receiving diabetes health information and education. Cardiovascular disease is prevalent in Type 2 diabetes due to a complex combination of various risk factors that trigger atherosclerosis – such as elevated blood fats, obesity and insulin resistance. Cardiovascular risk presents prior to a diagnosis of Type 2 diabetes, estimated to be up to 12 years before (Rydén, et al., 2013; Diabetes UK, 2008).

The enormity of diabetes, its complications and the need for vigilant and ongoing self-care can be a daunting prospect for the newly diagnosed, and often a depressing burden for individuals with long-duration diabetes. Stigma may have distinctly adverse effects on disease self-management (Skinner, et al., 2010; Sirey, et al., 2001a). However, there has never been a better time to be diagnosed with diabetes in terms of current technological advances, medical understanding of this condition and the help that is now available. As we have seen in earlier chapters however, according to personal circumstances, individuals may not engage fully in trying to manage their condition as effectively as possible.

The escalating prevalence of Type 2 diabetes

One in ten people over 40 in the UK are now living with a diagnosis of Type 2 diabetes: a total of 3.8 million people now have a diagnosis of diabetes in the UK, the large majority of those with Type 2 (Diabetes UK, 2019b). Type 2 diabetes usually occurs in individuals who are over the age of 40 (Diabetes UK, 2012b). However, the condition is increasingly being diagnosed in children and young adults. At any age, obesity, impaired glucose regulation, high blood fats, reduced high-density lipids, and hypertension can occur; glucose absorption by cells – stimulated by insulin – is then reduced. The major risk factor is obesity, counting for 80–85 percent of overall risk, underlying the current worldwide spread of Type 2 diabetes (Diabetes UK, 2012b). Whilst this is the case, obesity does not cause Type 2 diabetes and the condition also develops in those who are not obese due to other factors; conversely, obese individuals do not automatically develop Type 2 diabetes.

Both genetic and environmental factors increase the risk of developing Type 2, meaning that individuals who have close family members with the condition are 2–6 times more likely to develop Type 2 than the general population without this familial predisposition (Vaxilliare and Froguel, 2010). South Asian individuals are six times more likely to develop Type 2 diabetes – predominantly around age 25, while those of

Afro-Caribbean origin are three times more likely than Caucasian individuals to develop Type 2 diabetes (Department of Health, 2001).

Type 2 diabetes may develop very gradually because the symptoms – excessive urination and thirst, tiredness, blurred vision, slow healing of wounds, and numbness in the feet and legs – are far milder than in Type 1 diabetes. As Type 2 diabetes onset is slow, symptoms may go unrecognised or are tolerated by the individual for many years: the condition may only be detected during a routine blood test or visit to the doctor. However, complications of diabetes due to ongoing elevated blood glucose levels – such as eye, nerve or kidney disease – may have already begun before diabetes diagnosis. After diagnosis, there may be confusion and misunderstanding regarding the importance of managing the condition well.

Type 2 diabetes management

The number of people developing Type 2 diabetes is now so great that healthcare professionals in the UK cannot keep up with the volume of new diagnoses. The provision of information, education and support about diabetes assumes that the individual is enabled to manage their condition well, although this may not be the case in practice. The following comments are from individuals with Type 2 diabetes who have participated in DESMOND training – Diabetes Education and Self-Management for Ongoing and Newly Diagnosed. They suggest that a section of the Type 2 population has difficulty accepting and adjusting to their condition, having little understanding of what the condition involves, and poor knowledge and motivation to manage it as well as possible.

'I need extra sugar to boost my blood glucose with Type 2 diabetes. I only learnt this because a friend's child is Type 1 diabetic'.

'My GP told me to attend the DESMOND diabetes course. I was still suffering shock that I even had diabetes, but they didn't seem to understand that. The course was all about what I had to give up if I wanted to keep well and after about half an hour, I just walked out'.

'I often eat cakes and biscuits because life's too short to deny yourself all the time. I don't really understand why it matters, apart

> from that I might get heart disease one day. Well, I might get that
> anyway...'
>   'I have carbohydrate-intolerant diabetes'.

Conversely, individuals who had attended the DAFNE – Dosage Adjustment For Normal Eating – training for people with Type 1 diabetes had a far better understanding of why effective diabetes self-management is necessary.

> 'You have to give the right amount of insulin after assessing the carbohydrate content of food, not like when I just had two injections a day and had to watch what I ate. As the course says, dosage adjustment for NORMAL eating!'
>   'I actively try to minimise the risk of any complications by maintaining good blood glucose levels – it's important to look after yourself. I've got a friend with Type 2 who eats sweets regularly and doesn't care if she dies a bit earlier because of it, as long as she's enjoyed her life. I really can't understand why someone with diabetes would think like that'.

Information provision does not necessarily mean increased knowledge: understanding of a certain subject is derived from many sources. When that subject is diabetes, the individual may have friends and family with the condition, developing a perception of what it is like to live with the condition. The portrayal of diabetes for dramatic effect in films, television soap operas and books may give an inappropriate picture, although the media aims to educate viewers and readers about diabetes via a character. The individual's perception of what having diabetes involves, and how to cope with it, is therefore not just shaped by receiving an education message or leaflet from a diabetes clinic or GP surgery. Whilst it takes time to adjust to a diagnosis of diabetes, Type 2 diabetes might not be taken as seriously as Type 1.

> 'Type 2 diabetes – is that my sugar levels?'
>   'I take tablets for diabetes and then I can eat what I like. Sometimes, I feel unwell and have to lie down and have a sleep'.
>   'It's only Type 2 so it's not very serious'.
>   'I just ignore it because I don't think I've got diabetes'.

Obese individuals achieving poor blood glucose control with diet and exercise alone are prescribed Metformin diabetes medication, also prescribed for the same purpose without obesity. The gastrointestinal side-effects of Metformin can have a psychological impact on the individual due to diarrhoea and flatulence. The medication should also be used with caution for those with decreased kidney function, liver dysfunction and cardiac impairment. Annual monitoring of Type 2 diabetes should involve psychological assessment, especially for those with poor glycaemic control. A cardiovascular function and diabetes complications risk assessment is undertaken, as well as any management of blood fats, introducing statins to reduce cholesterol levels. Anti-thrombotic treatment, such as a daily 75mg dose of aspirin helps to prevent blood clots.

Despite established guidelines for ongoing Type 2 diabetes checks, in January 2016 the UK Government announced that diabetes care was a post-code lottery in this respect, stating that huge variations exist in diabetes education, psychological support, care and management across the country. Since the Covid-19 pandemic began in early 2020, millions have been waiting over a year for routine hospital care, with waiting times now at a 12-year high in England (BBC, October, 2020). Ophthalmology appointments have been delayed for those with diabetes, whilst diabetes reviews have been conducted by telephone rather than in-person, meaning clinicians are unable to carry out eye, kidney and foot checks.

Type 2 is now so common, the two main types of diabetes are no longer differentiated by many healthcare professionals and the blanket term 'diabetes' is used to cover both types, it often being assumed that the individual has Type 2. Therefore, those with Type 1 diabetes of long-duration from childhood may find that they now need to explain this differentiation.

Additionally, whilst individuals know they have diabetes, some may be unaware if they have Type 1 or Type 2, as insulin is also necessary for the management of Type 2. With a poor understanding of the potential serious consequences of the condition if not properly managed and the importance of good self-care and ongoing healthcare appointments, healthcare professionals may find this challenging. Some individuals with Type 2 diabetes feel unfairly judged as a result:

'You take the tablets and feel OK, but I've been told you're not really. The nurse gets annoyed with me for not understanding'.

'I don't know if I've got Type 1 or Type 2. I didn't always have to, but now I inject twice a day and drink a lot of Lucozade because I'm a manual worker and often feel unwell. That's all I know. My doctor says I don't listen'.

'I think it's Type 2, but I know I feel sick if I eat sweets or doughnuts. The diabetes nurse just shakes her head when I say that'.

Type 2 diabetes management is designed to meet the individual's needs with a care plan tailored to specific glucose difficulties and any additional health conditions (National Institute for Health and Care Excellence, 2014a). The plan includes nutritional advice, where a higher HbA1c target may be set as management with diet alone means glucose levels cannot be reduced with tablets or insulin. Although NICE recommends a diabetes management plan tailored to specific glucose irregularities, the individual's understanding of their condition may mean this plan is not followed, being perceived as overwhelming, ultimately translating into denial or poor motivation for self-care.

'A close family member has Type 1 diabetes, but doesn't look after it properly. When I developed Type 2, I knew it wasn't as bad as hers, so I do the same as she does because I don't really want to know'.

'I don't read things about diabetes because it just depresses me. Years ago, I decided that if I don't know I can't worry about it, then it doesn't seem like such a big deal'.

'Type 2 diabetes is not going to ruin my life. I eat and drink what I like, when I like as it's too much hassle to be dieting and worrying about how many carbohydrates I'm having or whether I'm doing enough exercise. I've never had a hypo, so I must be doing OK'.

The tightrope walk of Type 2 and exercise

Many individuals are taught to manage Type 2 diabetes with a carbohydrate-restricted diet and regular exercise when the condition is first diagnosed. However, the individual may not be told about the complex relationship between glucose and exercise. Intense exercise can cause the liver to release glucose stored as glucagon, raising blood glucose levels; it is a common misconception that exercise automatically burns and lowers glucose levels. Response to exercise depends on how much blood glucose is already present because glucose is the sole fuel for muscles. Intense exercise initiates a seven to eightfold increase in glucose production, while glucose utilisation only rises three to fourfold (Marliss and Vranic, 2002).

Glucose utilisation is dependent on regulating influences such as insulin, plasma glucose and muscle factors. A rise in glucose availability occurs when exercise is undertaken and this response cannot be avoided, even with the administration of additional insulin − not always prescribed for those with Type 2. When the stage of exhaustion is reached following intense exercise, there is substantial hyperglycaemia because more glucose is available than is needed. For an individual without diabetes, the pancreas produces more insulin for 40–60 minutes after intense exercise while blood glucose levels are high, but this natural insulin response is absent in diabetes, causing sustained hyperglycaemia if additional insulin or diabetes medication is not taken. Exercise-induced hyperglycaemia is therefore commonly reported by individuals with diabetes (Marliss and Vranic, 2002).

Moderate exercise reduces blood glucose, but if levels are initially above 15mmol/L, or 270mg/dl, it is not advisable to exercise − high blood glucose levels exert undue strain on the heart. Conversely, hypoglycaemia may occur if too much insulin is administered and exercise is taken; exercise increases insulin mobilisation from the site at which it is administered so that more is working at one time, particularly if the exercised region − e.g., arm, is the same as the administration site (Marliss and Vranic, 2002). The risk of hypoglycemia depends on the pre-exercise blood glucose level: the rise in working insulin blocks the effect glucagon has on glucose production by the liver. This also increases glucose utilisation to a higher degree than is necessary for the exercise (Marliss and Vranic, 2002).

'My doctor and friends think I don't try to manage my Type 2. Actually, I do two sessions in the gym each week but because I'm only prescribed tablets, my bloods are always high afterwards and I have no way to lower them again. I told the diabetes nurse and she didn't believe I was exercising – she said that exercise would lower my blood glucose levels, not increase them, so I was wrong. I then get blamed for having a high HbA1c and not sticking to my diabetes plan. It's very de-motivating and the "experts" don't seem equipped to help. I enjoy the exercise and social contact at the gym sessions as it makes me feel good mentally, so I don't want to give it up'.

Type 2 diabetes reversal with diet and exercise

Dietary changes alone have little effect on Type 2 diabetes, although with lifestyle change in addition to weight loss, it is possible to reverse glucose impairment in obese individuals (Ahmad and Crandall, 2010). A behavioural change approach to reversing Type 2 diabetes has been documented since the late 1990s (Holford, 2011; Boden, et al., 2005; Harder, et al., 2004; Vernon, et al., 2003). In the United States, an intensive lifestyle change intervention involving calorie, carbohydrate and fat restriction successfully prevented Type 2 diabetes in obese in-dividuals at high risk of developing the condition (Mayer-Davis, et al., 2004).

Other research studies suggest similar findings. Westman, et al. (2008) reported that 85 individuals with Type 2 diabetes eating <20 g daily carbohydrate for six months but no calorie restriction achieved reduced blood glucose levels and improved HbA1c levels. Carbohydrates – starches – are converted to glucose, so low-carbohydrate diets are also low glycaemic index diets, stabilising blood glucose increases. By eliminating or strictly reducing carbohydrate intake, the need for dia-betes medication to manage glucose levels is reduced. This evidence suggests that lifestyle change can reverse Type 2 diabetes if health im-provement is a motivating factor for the individual.

A calorie-restricted diet is not the same as healthy eating and/or redu-cing carbohydrate intake as low-carbohydrate diets may permit a normal fat intake – meaning they are not low-calorie. Rapid weight loss may be required for the individual to undergo surgery, where <800 calories a day is necessary. These restrictive diets can lead to vitamin and mineral deficiency and are only undertaken for three months under medical supervision (NICE, 2014c). If the individual has Type 2 diabetes and reduced liver or kidney function, cardiac impairment, disordered eating and other psychological health issues, a restricted diet may not be suitable.

> 'Sessions with a dietician and psychologist helped me see I was comfort eating. Once I understood the root cause, I realised I was just eating for the sake of it and not because of actual hunger. I know this sounds simple, but I've managed to lose 20kg and now my Type 2 diabetes levels are normal'.
>
> 'Things happened in my life that I felt were my fault: I was in care homes for a lot of my childhood. I never connected this with my enjoyment of food and paid to see a counsellor until it clicked into place and made sense. Every time I wanted junk food I reminded myself of what we'd discussed. My diabetes consultant hopes I can eventually come off Metformin completely as I've lost weight and feel so much better'.

Current recommendations from the National Institute for Care Excellence (NICE, 2014c) suggest that gastric band surgery enabling weight loss should be offered to more individuals with Type 2 diabetes to reduce the annual cost of treating diabetes; in 2019, Diabetes UK estimated this to be 14 billion pounds every year (Diabetes UK, 2019c). Whilst dietary restriction and exercise may not be suitable for morbidly obese individuals, lifestyle change has fewer complications and side-effects than surgery and is cheaper for the NHS. Adopting a lifestyle change for weight loss requires motivation and support from healthcare professionals. The issues underlying overeating need to be investigated and addressed to achieve success.

Excess body fat blocks the action of insulin on the cells, leading to insulin resistance and increased blood glucose levels. Fat loss allows insulin to work normally, improving glycaemic control in obese individuals with Type 2 diabetes. This can mean glucose-reducing medication is no longer necessary. A modified diet and regular cardiovascular exercise has the potential to revert to a pre-diabetes state without the side-effects of bariatric surgery. However, changing eating patterns has physical and psychological implications: a weight loss plan must be tailored to the individual's specific needs by appropriately trained health professionals offering ongoing assistance and support. Weight loss surgery or diet and exercise are not quick-fix solutions as adopted lifestyle changes must become permanent, requiring the individual to be highly motivated to succeed.

Type 2 diabetes reversal with weight loss surgery

Defined as a Body Mass Index – BMI – of >30 kg/m^2, obesity is a chronic condition that is rapidly escalating in adults and children. Obesity is now a worldwide pandemic (Berry, 2020), being a significant risk factor for many health conditions including heart disease; Type 2 diabetes; hypertension; dyslipidemia; stroke; atheroscleroisis – fatty deposits in the arteries, and certain cancers (Whitlock, et al., 2009). As well as being a risk factor for serious physical disease, obesity also leads to psychological disorders, disordered eating and an impaired quality of life for the individual with complications, mortality increasing with the duration of obesity (Kubik, et al., 2013). Morbid obesity – defined as a BMI of above 40 kg/m^2 – is now frequently seen.

The National Institute for Health and Care Excellence have estimated that more than 25 percent of UK adults are now classed as obese and a further 42 percent of men and a third of women are overweight, whilst 1 in 6 NHS beds is taken up by a person with Type 1 or Type 2 diabetes and complications (NICE, 2014b). Almost 2 million morbidly obese individuals could benefit from bariatric surgery, potentially reversing 40,000 cases of Type 2 diabetes and 5,000 cases of heart disease as currently, 17 billion pounds each year is spent by the NHS on obesity-related conditions.

The full extent of the psychological effects of obesity is unclear, although weight loss of 5–10 percent is beneficial in ameliorating chronic health conditions that are exacerbated by excess body fat (Obesity Health Alliance, 2017). Whilst adopting a healthy lifestyle and moderate exercise is successful for the mild to moderately overweight, this approach is inadvisable for the morbidly obese. Bariatric surgery – fitting a gastric band to drastically reduce the size of the stomach – is challenging for the individual, who must make significant changes to diet and exercise behaviour as well as lifestyle in order for the surgery to be successful. Some individuals, however, will continue to binge eat (Niego, et al., 2007).

'After surgery, I only managed to stick to the restricted diet for about a month. Then I began to cheat with lots of ice cream and full-fat coffees because I felt miserable, so I actually put the 10 pounds I'd lost back on, plus a bit more. Eventually, I had to admit what I'd been doing. My doctor threatened to remove the band if I wasn't going to use it properly. I felt so guilty and ashamed that it forced me to be good'.

'It's so hard, going without the foods you love. Yes, I want to be thinner, but I wasn't prepared for how low I'd feel all the time. At least when I could eat, I was happy. Who wants to be thin and miserable?'

Bariatric surgery restricts the quantity of food that can be eaten and reduces the amount of nutrients that can be absorbed. There are two kinds of bariatric procedure: restrictive surgeries and malabsorptive/restrictive surgeries. Restrictive surgeries work by reducing the size of the stomach to slow down digestion so the individual stays fuller for longer with less food. Malabsorptive/restrictive surgeries are more invasive and involve physically removing a portion of the digestive tract to restrict calorie absorption.

One example of restrictive surgery involves placing a synthetic band around the upper portion of the stomach to form a small pouch just below the oesophagus, significantly reducing the quantity of food consumed and cutting calories. The size of the pouch can be surgically altered by inflating or deflating the band through an implanted port beneath the skin on the abdomen: the band can be removed at any time. Alternative procedures include laparoscopic sleeve gastrectomy – where part of the stomach is sectioned off so that less food is needed to become full, and biliopancreatic diversion – surgery to reduce the size of the stomach and intestine to limit food intake and absorption.

The reversal of Type 2 diabetes in morbidly obese individuals was first observed more than 10 years ago following bariatric surgery (Keidar, 2011). Certain procedures, such as the Roux-en-Y gastric bypass (RYGBP) and biliopancreatic diversion (BPD), are more effective treatments for the reversal of Type 2 diabetes than traditional weight loss or medication. These methods have been particularly successful in returning levels of plasma glucose, insulin and HbA1c to normal levels in 80–100 percent of morbidly obese individuals (Keidar, 2011). However, surgery results in a loss of life expectancy for those with extremely high BMIs over 60 kg/m² (Schauer, et al., 2015).

Remarkably, normal blood glucose and insulin levels return only days after surgery, even though there has been no significant weight loss (Rubiano, et al., 2010; 2006a, 2006b, Schernthaner and Morton, 2008; Crookes, 2006). This suggests that insulin is able to work more effectively due to factors other than weight loss alone, such as decreased food intake, reduced malabsorption of nutrients, and anatomical change in the gastrointestinal tract affecting glucose metabolism. A greater understanding of these mechanisms may lead to new treatments for Type 2 diabetes and obesity in the future. Behaviour change interventions have targeted healthy eating and regular exercise to tackle obesity with the addition of weight loss medication. Any significant weight loss has rarely been achieved, especially by the morbidly obese as they do not restrict their eating, with a failure rate of around 95 percent at one year (Tsai and Wadden, 2005; Buchwald, 2004).

Successful reversal of Type 2 diabetes has been reported, involving discontinuation of medication and the achievement of normal blood glucose levels in up to 86.6 percent of individuals (Keidar, 2011; Buchwald, 2005). Following bariatric surgery there was an average weight loss of 38.5 kilograms, equating to almost 56 percent of excess weight (Buchwald, et al., 2009). Further research involving 240 morbidly obese individuals following bariatric surgery reported that 80 percent became diabetes-free, with an average weight loss of 60 percent – 44kg (Schauer, et al., 2003). Individuals with a <5-year duration of Type 2 diabetes who could formerly control blood glucose levels with diet alone achieved the best weight loss and were more likely to have their diabetes reversed by bariatric surgery.

Research has compared morbidly obese individuals with a <2-year duration of conventionally-managed Type 2 diabetes to those following bariatric surgery. Results showed significant reductions in fasting blood glucose, HbA1c and the need for diabetes medication (Dixon, et al., 2008). A further 10-year follow-up of 268 individuals found that 97 percent of participants sustained normal blood glucose and HbA1c levels for that decade (Marinari, et al., 2006). These studies show that the reversal of Type 2 diabetes following bariatric surgery can achieve long-term outcomes, significantly reducing mortality as a result. Deaths attributed to Type 2 diabetes are reduced by 92 percent, proving unequivocally that weight loss surgery is an extremely effective treatment for the condition (Adams, et al., 2007). This success rate has prompted the use of bariatric procedures as a worldwide treatment option for Type 2 diabetes where there is morbid obesity and overweight.

Potential complications of weight loss surgery

Complications arising from bariatric surgery vary according to the type of procedure (Crookes, 2006). Simpler gastric banding restrictive procedures are less invasive and rarely affect bowel function, equating to a reduced risk of nutrient malabsorption and subsequent vitamin deficiency unless there is repeated vomiting. There is potential for band erosion from hydrochloric stomach acid and digestive enzymes, resulting in abdominal pain and diminished weight loss (Keidar, 2011). Over-expansion of the band has resulted in band slippage, effectively making the food pouch larger with either no weight loss or weight gain being reported (Crookes, et al., 2008; Keidar, et al., 2005).

Surgical procedures to restrict the absorption of nutrients can lead to major dietary deficiencies. In the first month following bariatric surgery there may be poor wound healing – a particular problem in those with diabetes, and incision hernias – pushing part of the digestive tract out of its normal position – following bypass and re-joining parts of the small bowel to reduce nutrient absorption (Podnos, et al., 2003). Small bowel obstruction has been reported in 2.1 percent of individuals, and narrowing of the small bowel in 0.7 percent of surgeries; gastrointestinal bleeding in 0.6 percent following surgery; leakage of the contents of the small bowel at the surgery site in 1.2 percent; blockage of the pulmonary artery by a blood clot – pulmonary embolus – in 1.0 percent of cases, and pneumonia in 0.1–0.3 percent of individuals following gastric bypass procedures (Keidar, 2011).

Later-onset complications of gastric bypass concern the disruptive effect of surgery on the gastro-intestinal tract. Nutritional deficiencies are a major concern, especially the potential lack of protein-calories – resulting in swelling of the lower limbs and a feeling of weakness; calcium and iron depletion and vitamin deficiencies. This emphasises the need for excellent nutrition in the much-reduced portion sizes with the addition of appropriate vitamin supplementation. In this context, Schweiger, et al. (2010) state that nutritional deficiencies can develop as a result of anorexia; prolonged vomiting; poor vitamin and mineral supplementation and stricture formation, the growth of scar tissue causing narrowing; or malabsorption of nutrients.

'I thought weight loss surgery would help me be slim and healthy. Instead, I ended up with nerve damage due to vitamin deficiencies, gallstones and terrible heartburn, chronic constipation, tremendous pain and headaches. I've felt anxious every day since

> the surgery, and so depressed that it's all been such a nightmare – and this is what I signed up for, so I've only got myself to blame. Yes, I've lost some weight, but now I've got so many health problems, it just wasn't worth it'.

Severe vitamin deficiency may occur following weight loss surgery due to continual vomiting (Berger, 2004). Such deficiencies cause neurological complications, such as beri-beri – a lack of vitamin B1. Wet beri-beri affects the heart and circulatory system, while dry beri-beri affects the nerves and reduces muscle strength. Wernicke's encephalopathy – a neurological disorder caused by vitamin B1 deficiency – may also occur. Peripheral neuropathy, commonly associated with diabetes, is a potential complication of bariatric surgery, as are spinal cord lesions due to vitamin B12 and folic acid deficiency. Iron and calcium deficiency due to a reduced absorption in the duodenum and jejunum frequently occurs in females of child-bearing age following this procedure (Coates, et al., 2004; Skroubis, et al., 2002). Loss of bone density is a consequence of calcium deficiency following gastric bypass surgery, and vitamin D deficiency – essential for a healthy immune system and bone strength in association with calcium – may go undetected as deficiency results in generalised muscle pain and weakness.

Heartburn and regurgitation have been reported in those who have undergone malabsorptive/restrictive surgeries (Keidar, et al., 2010; Crookes, et al., 2006). Due to the nature of the surgery, bowel disturbances are commonly experienced by patients following weight loss procedures, although the body adapts to this change over time. When the surgery is restrictive rather than also malabsorptive, constipation may result due to a reduced volume of food passing through the digestive tract with less fibre content. The formation of gallstones – cholelithiasis – is also a common complication of rapid weight loss for any reason (Keidar, 2011; Crookes, 2006).

Type 2 diabetes and surgery risks

For those with Type 2 diabetes, bariatric surgery is a serious undertaking, increasing the chance of morbidity and mortality following this procedure. Microvascular changes associated with diabetes lead to poor blood supply, meaning that wound healing is slow. This is a primary reason for leakage and associated complications following procedures involving open and laparoscopic methods – via a small incision into the abdominal cavity (Fernandez, et al., 2004). However, the need to achieve weight loss via a reduced intake of food to reverse Type 2 diabetes outweighs the surgical mortality and morbidity risk. A 92 percent reduction in deaths from Type 2 diabetes following reversal of the condition by gastric bypass has been documented (Adams, 2007).

The National Institute for Health and Care Excellence (NICE, 2014b; 2014c) advises that obese individuals with recently diagnosed Type 2 diabetes should be offered weight loss surgery if they have a BMI of over 35. Although there is an initial cost to the NHS of around £6,000 per procedure, in the long-term the cost of treating Type 2 diabetes and its complications – including anxiety and depression – would be far greater. Therefore, by employing surgical treatment of Type 2 diabetes before complications arise from prolonged hyperglycaemia, the individual can achieve a better quality of life. The need to prevent complications is demonstrated below.

'I funded my own weight loss surgery a couple of years ago. I took insulin for Type 2 diabetes and, almost immediately, my sugar levels were normal without insulin injections, even though I hadn't lost much weight. Unfortunately, I already had eye and nerve problems that haven't improved or gone away, despite my blood sugar and HbA1c being normal. This has been very distressing'.

'After a heart attack, I had a gastric band fitted last year. I've lost weight and my diabetes has actually gone, but it was years before my diabetes was properly diagnosed, causing damage to my heart and circulation that can't be reversed'.

Gastric bypass surgery to treat obesity and Type 2 diabetes is known to reduce diabetes-related deaths by up to 90 percent (Scopinaro, et al., 2005). It is clear that those with morbid obesity and Type 2 diabetes can benefit from surgical intervention, although mortality risk requires discussion in order for the individual to make an informed decision about going ahead with the procedure. An average 47.5 percent of total bodyweight is lost with a gastric band and 61.6 percent for those undergoing gastric bypass surgery (Buchwald, et al., 2009). A plateau of weight loss is reached at around two years following surgery, and there may be some weight gain in the third year (Sarwer, et al., 2012). Bariatric surgery leads to the significant improvement of various weight-related health conditions in addition to Type 2 diabetes: metabolic syndrome and an early death from cardiac risk factors can also be reversed (Dixon, et al., 2008; O'Brien, et al., 2006, Sjöström, et al., 1999). Weight loss procedures offer a cost-effective solution to morbid obesity before the individual develops comorbidities (Picot, et al., 2009)

Weight loss surgery for children with Type 2 diabetes

Increasing rates of extreme obesity in children are associated with not only Type 2 diabetes but also other 'adult onset' diseases, such as obstructive sleep apnoea; fatty liver disease – steatohepatitis, and heart disease, with severely obese adolescents being particularly vulnerable (Kubik, et al., 2013). Children and young adults with obesity are known to experience significant alienation, low self-esteem, body dissatisfaction, depressive symptoms, poor control of eating behaviour, harmful weight control behaviours – such as anorexia and/or bulimia nervosa, and impaired social relationships (Vander Wal and Mitchell, 2011; Zeller, et al., 2011; 2006). The level of weight-related distress increases with age and is worse in girls than in boys (Erickskson, et al., 2000). Research assessing quality of life experienced by obese children and adolescents showed similar findings to young persons diagnosed with cancer (Schwimmer, et al., 2003).

Childhood obesity is often related to poor family understanding of nutrition and portion control, so the whole family must become involved in tackling the problem. This type of approach relies on health education concerning the family reducing calories and increasing the amount of regular exercise (Barlow, 2007). Kubik, et al. (2013) suggest that this approach is rarely successful on its own, although when combined with weight loss medication, this situation improves (Chanoine, et al., 2005).

Bariatric surgery is only considered for young adults with life-threatening obesity in extreme cases where the need outweighs the risk. The success rate of such procedures in adolescents is similar to that in adults, with 40–60 percent of excess weight lost in the first year and >75 percent by the end of the second year, (Kubik, et al., 2013; Hsia, et al., 2012). In such cases, a long-term risk assessment is undertaken (Hsia, et al., 2012).

In adults and adolescents undergoing weight loss surgery, there is normalised or significantly improved blood pressure, insulin resistance, Type 2 diabetes and levels of blood fats. Following stomach restriction/ malabsorption procedures, levels of depression, anxiety and self-perception are reported to improve after as little as four months

(Jarvholm, et al., 2012), and is still present after four years (Zeller, et al., 2011). Mental health is therefore strongly correlated with weight control although positive outcomes were reported before any significant weight loss, suggesting that the surgery offers a perceived improved quality of life.

> 'I had my stomach stapled when I was 16 because my diabetes doctor thought it would improve my sugar levels with Type 2 diabetes. It was really hard, not joining in with friends who were going to McDonalds or Pizza Hut, but a couple of close friends were supportive. I've lost a steady but small amount of weight and I'm now really hopeful for the future as my weight won't hold me back'.

Significant physical and psychological benefits can be achieved for young and adult individuals following weight loss surgery. The benefit of undergoing a surgical procedure must outweigh any potential short and long-term risks as obesity is driven by eating disorders; the individual may not experience remission of psychological symptoms following surgery. Weight loss surgery enables a level of hope, expectation and perceived control over both obesity and life issues. However, the individual may have unrealistic expectations that weight loss surgery will miraculously solve every problem they face, with the reality potentially being difficult to accept.

The psychological impact of weight loss surgery

Surgery to achieve weight loss can successfully treat a number of health problems such as morbid obesity and Type 2 diabetes; reversal of diabetes also stabilises chronic and life-threatening complications of the disease. When both weight loss and diabetes reversal is achieved, the surgery is considered to have been effective, but in the light of this success the individual is forced to adopt considerable behavioural change affecting their perception of wellbeing, despite psychological counselling.

'I was advised to have weight loss surgery to help my diabetes. It sounded like an easy solution because I've always struggled with my weight and health. Although the risks were explained, it didn't sink in – possible death doesn't seem real when you're sitting in the consultant's office, nodding at everything you're being told. I just wanted to lose weight and feel better. After the operation, I was very ill with a long stay in hospital. If I'd known this from experience rather than just being told, I would still have gone ahead, but I didn't realise how hard life would be without the pleasure of food as it's part of every occasion. I miss that, even though my diabetes has gone because I've lost 33kg'.

Although the physical complications of bariatric surgery are widely documented, the psychological implications are less so. It is known that morbidly obese individuals experience mood disorders, anxiety and low self-esteem and are five times more likely to have suffered major depression in the previous five years than average weight individuals (Sarwer, et al., 2012). Depression is common among morbidly obese individuals for several reasons; for women especially, a major factor is body dissatisfaction due to pressure to conform to societal norms (Kubik, et al., 2013). Obesity also carries stigma, causing prejudice and discrimination, leading to or worsening depression (Arora, et al., 2019; Sikorski, et al., 2011).

Evidence suggests that morbid obesity equates to poorer socio-economic status regarding lower household income, lesser educational achievement, and a greater likelihood of being single when compared with average weight peers with a similar intellect (Kubik, et al., 2013). Depressive symptoms are further intensified by yo-yo dieting where weight loss attempts fail, heightening feelings of hopelessness and low self-esteem (Wooley and Garner, 1991).

Depressive symptoms due to the factors of body image, low self-esteem and stigma contribute to the complex decision to proceed with surgery; this has been reported by 20–30 percent of individuals before they undertake bariatric procedures, with 50 percent citing a life-long history of depression (Sarwer, et al., 2012). The psychological health of obese individuals is strongly correlated with further weight gain.

Individuals undergoing bariatric surgery are more likely to experience psychological distress compared with obese persons who do not have these procedures (Abiles, et al., 2010). The trigger to self-initiate bariatric surgery rather than it being advised by a physician is frequently due to a distressing or traumatic event, such as the death of a loved one (Kalarchian, et al., 2007). Similarly, those seeking surgical or medication-based solutions to obesity are more likely to have experienced psychological distress than those requesting dietary advice and behavioural therapy for their obesity (Higgs, et al., 1997). Poor mental health has also been attributed to individuals with Type 2 diabetes in association with obesity (Anderson, et al., 2001; Dew, 1998). The impact of living with complications such as diabetes-related heart disease, blindness, kidney disease, and/or nerve pain takes a massive toll on the individual physically and mentally.

To be eligible for NHS bariatric surgery, the individual must have failed to lose weight with diet and exercise and have a BMI of >40, or a BMI of above 35 if there is also an obesity-related comorbidity such as Type 2 diabetes (Kubik, et al., 2013). Although expensive and potentially life-threatening, the surgery aims to achieve and maintain substantial weight loss. Surgery to reduce the amount of food that can be eaten forces the individual to completely change eating and exercise habits. Selection of suitable candidates for weight loss surgery involves in-depth assessment of medical, psychological and social issues.

'They asked me everything, basically to assess if I was a stable person who could handle the surgery and go without much food for the rest of my life. I admit that I lied about my mental health to get them to agree to the surgery. Months later, I now find it extremely hard to just eat very small meals for their nutrition content – I actually resent good food because I HAVE to eat it rather than because I want it, and I desperately miss cakes and biscuits. The cravings for 'nice' comfort food haven't left me and I'm so depressed now'.

Research and comprehensive reviews suggest that weight loss surgery leads to higher self-esteem, improved depressive symptoms, health-related quality of life, and a more positive body image (Van Hout, 2006; Van Hout, et al., 2005; Bocchieri, et al., 2002). There is generally a good adaptation to behaviour change and a substantial decrease in depression and anxiety in the year following the procedure compared to those undergoing counselling, diet and exercise alone. It is clear that these mental health benefits come as a result of the individual's weight loss following bariatric surgery; any reported post-operative weight regain is associated with an increase in depressive symptoms (Bocchieri, et al., 2002).

Depression and anxiety are common in morbidly obese individuals Research suggests that psychological issues can be attributed to obesity rather than personality, meaning that improvements in psychological health may be due to the amount of weight lost (Mamplekou, et al., 2005; Guisado, et al., 2002). However, psychological health benefits are also seen in those who do not lose any weight following bariatric surgery and before the desired outcome of surgery has occurred (Dymek, et al., 2001). Higgs, et al (1997) suggest that undergoing bariatric surgery lifts the burden of the distressing event triggering the desire for a surgical solution to life-threatening obesity. Positive mental health effects are therefore due to a proactive attitude to tackle obesity, despite little or no weight loss.

Despite the ability of bariatric surgery to reverse or improve overall physical and mental health status, a minority of individuals do not view this surgery as a positive way forward. Van Hout (2006) and Bocchieri, et al. (2002) have reported a reduction in long-term health, or no obvious benefit following weight loss surgery. There may be unrealistic expectations of dramatic changes following weight loss surgery, effectively setting the individual up for disappointment. If these expectations are not met, this has a negative impact on mental health, even with significant weight loss; those who have undergone bariatric procedures may realise that they cannot attribute underlying emotional disturbance to their weight. Additionally, some individuals may have difficulty coping with negative life events that they are no longer able to attribute to their obesity.

'After my surgery, I stupidly thought life would be different because the weight would be gone. I thought that I'd be more popular and have a fantastic social life – that being thin would change everything. In reality, my life is exactly the same except I'm no longer fat. It's the same life and the same problems – looking after my elderly mother and a lack of support from others. While I've got more confidence now to get a better job and make a better life, I was expecting too much from the surgery and now I'm just as miserable'.

Any reduction in depressive symptoms following bariatric surgery does not last. Sanchez-Zaldıvar, et al. (2009) reported decreasing levels of depression for a period of two years following surgery; whilst a depression-free post-operative period of four years has been suggested by Frigg, et al. (2004). Some improvement in depressive symptoms followed by subsequent decline has also been observed, associated with weight loss followed by weight gain, or the individual reaching a plateau where no further weight is lost (Kubik, et al., 2013; Bocchieri, et al., 2002).

A key factor in boosting mental health following bariatric surgery is positive reinforcement gained through health professional interaction during post-operative appointments. This may explain why depressive symptoms re-appear with the reduced need for follow-up clinic visits over time. Mitchell, et al. (2013) and Peterhansel, et al. (2013) have reported completed suicide among individuals following weight loss surgery, although it is difficult to attribute this as the direct cause and it is unclear whether rates of suicide in such individuals are any higher than those of the general population. The potential risk for suicide highlights the necessity of ongoing assessment of mental health status, even though physical symptoms, such as raised blood glucose levels, may no longer be present.

The issue of self-concept

Self-concept is the individual's self-perception, shaped by characteristics such as self-esteem, body image and self-confidence, as well as perception of attractiveness and assertiveness. It is difficult to study these subjective factors because they are unique to the individual, but the personality shaped by these self-concepts can be observed. Available literature suggests that bariatric surgery increases self-esteem, self-confidence, and personality as a result of improved body image and weight loss satisfaction (Bocchieri, et al., 2002). Kubik, et al., (2013) report that 90 percent of individuals are pleased with their overall appearance following surgery, expressing increased satisfaction with body image despite minimal weight loss – meaning less loose skin: this being the greatest reason for dissatisfaction in those who had lost more weight. Kinzl, et al., (2013) reported similarly that 70 percent of those who have undergone bariatric surgery experienced significant distress and body image dissatisfaction because excess skin does not shrink in association with weight loss.

'I didn't realise there would be so much baggy skin hanging down. When I complained, the doctor explained that my skin had been stretched by the fat and wouldn't spring back naturally. I've lost weight but my body is still ugly. I'm having surgery to remove the skin on the underside of my arms soon. Then I'll get a date to have my legs done, a tummy tuck and bottom lift. I'm wondering when it will ever end. At the end of the day I'll have horrible long scars everywhere rather than the body I've always dreamed of.

'I wanted the problem to be fixed when I woke up after the surgery – that the fat would be gone and I would look normal and be confident. Like a personality transplant…'

These comments highlight that the individual must be prepared for a long journey following significant weight loss rather than a quick fix, although being told what to expect may not equate to full understanding. Showing anonymous photographs in order to convey the reality of loose skin following extreme weight loss may enable the individual to relate to this problem. Despite psychological counselling regarding post-operative effects of weight loss surgery, the individual must unfortunately learn by experience, potentially leading to dissatisfaction.

Plastic surgeons who carry out body contouring to remove excess skin are an important part of the counselling team, being in the ideal position to raise awareness of the limitations of this procedure. Adverse outcomes may not be in line with the individual's expectations and it is also difficult to assess any future personality traits. Van Hout, et al. (2006) reported an increased discipline following bariatric surgery, along with reduced neuroticism, defensiveness and immature identity. However, Kubik, et al. (2013) suggested that ingrained, long-duration personality traits were resistant to change post-surgery.

It is known that disordered eating, especially binge eating, is common in obese individuals, thought to occur in 5–15 percent of those who have had bariatric surgery (Sarwer, 2012). It is difficult to evaluate the extent of binge eating because it relies on self-reporting, as well as the under-reporting in studies of the subject, meaning the assessment of whether weight loss surgery can resolve binge eating remains uncertain. Van Hout, et al., (2006) suggest that binge eating behaviour is likely to be reversed following surgery as emphasis is then placed on dietary restriction. However, whilst eating a large quantity of calorific foods may be unachievable with a very small stomach size, intake of low-nutrition, high-fat foods such as ice cream can reduce weight loss or lead to weight gain.

While stating that bariatric surgery can be effective in reversing binge eating behaviour, Sarwer, et al., (2012) also suggest that many individuals continue with 'disturbing eating disorders' post-surgery such as exerting tight control over what is eaten for fear of weight gain. Some individuals report a loss of control over their eating and still feel the desire to overeat, deterred only by the surgical inability and the likelihood of vomiting if the stomach becomes over-full (Kubik, et al., 2013). Further research examining eating behaviour two years after bariatric surgery showed that some individuals used vomiting – effectively bulimia – to maintain their new weight and shape (de Zwaan, et al., 2010). This insight suggests that vomiting is self-induced and that such individuals are suffering from a significant eating disorder.

Key messages in this chapter:

- Cardiovascular risk presents prior to a diagnosis of Type 2 diabetes, estimated to be as long as 12 years before.
- Obesity counts for 80–85 percent of overall risk underlying the current worldwide increase in Type 2 diabetes. Obesity does not cause Type 2 diabetes and the condition also develops in the non-obese due to other factors. Conversely, obese individuals do not automatically develop Type 2 diabetes.
- Intense exercise can cause the liver to release stored glucose, raising blood glucose levels; it is a common misconception that exercise automatically lowers glucose levels as this relies on exercise intensity. Response to exercise also depends on how much glucose is already present because glucose is the sole fuel for muscles.
- Dietary changes alone have little effect on Type 2 diabetes, although with lifestyle change in addition to weight loss, it is possible to reverse glucose impairment in obese individuals.
- As well as being a risk factor for serious physical disease, obesity also leads to psychological disorders, disordered eating and an impaired quality of life for the individual, with complications and mortality increasing with the duration of obesity.
- The use of bariatric procedures is a worldwide treatment option for Type 2 diabetes where there is morbid obesity and overweight.
- There may be unrealistic expectations of dramatic and immediate changes following weight loss surgery, effectively setting the individual up for disappointment.

- Increasing rates of extreme obesity in children are associated with Type 2 diabetes; obstructive sleep apnoea; fatty liver disease, and heart disease, with severely obese adolescents being particularly vulnerable.
- Children and young adults with obesity experience significant alienation; low self-esteem; body dissatisfaction; depressive symptoms; poor control of eating behaviour; harmful weight control behaviours – such as anorexia and/or bulimia nervosa, and impaired social relationships.

Glossary of Terms

Adipose: fat tissue.

Acrocyanosis: intolerance to cold manifesting as bluish skin discolouration on the fingers, nose and ears due to poor circulation.

Acute adrenocortical hypofunction: (also called Addison's crisis or adrenal crisis) which is a medical emergency. It occurs due to a sudden reduction in hydrocortisone.

Addison's disease: (also known as chronic cortical hypofunction or adrenocortical insufficiency) develops due to slow destruction of the adrenal cortex due to autoimmune attack.

Adipokines: are produced by fat cells and are known to cause Type 2 diabetes, high blood pressure and narrowing of the arteries.

Adiponectin: hormone produced by the fat cells that causes the tissues to be sensitive to insulin.

Adrenal insufficiency: an alternative name for Addison's disease. A condition where there is reduced hormone production due to auto-immune damage reducing the release of hormones such as cortisol.

Aldosterone: a hormone secreted by the adrenal glands which acts to increase the uptake of sodium and the secretion of potassium.

ALT: Alanine Transaminase.

Amygdala: the part of the brain responsible for generating negative emotions.

Androgens: sex hormones.

Anorexia nervosa: where there is an obsessive fear of gaining weight resulting in severe dietary restriction.

Anterior cingulated cortex: the area of the brain responsible for attention, self-awareness and regulation.

Anti-atherogenic medications: reduce fatty deposits in the artery walls.

Anti-hypertensive drugs: reduce blood pressure.

Anti-neoplasticdrugs: prevent abnormal tissue growth.

AST: Aspartate Transaminase.

Atheroma: pertaining to atherosclerosis – fatty deposits in the arteries causing narrowing and arterial disease.

Atherosclerosis: a degenerative disease of the arteries associated with fatty deposits on the inner walls leading to reduced blood flow.

Autoimmune diseases: chronic health conditions such as Type 1 diabetes, where the disease is caused by immune system attack.

Autoimmune hepatitis: an autoimmune disorder when the immune system attacks the liver cells, causing inflammation.

Bariatric surgery: where a gastric band is fitted or a small pouch created by dividing the stomach so that calorie intake is drastically reduced.

Basal rate: in terms of insulin pump therapy this is the set amount of background insulin delivered per hour to maintain blood glucose levels within normal limits.

Behaviour Change Wheel: developed from 19 frameworks of behaviour change identified in a systematic literature review, the hub identifies sources of the behaviour that could be targets for intervention. It uses the COM-B ('capability', 'opportunity', 'motivation' and 'behaviour') model.

Beri-beri: vitamin B1 deficiency which can be either dry, causing heart and circulatory problems, or wet, causing neurological problems accompanied by muscle weakness.

BDI: Beck Depression Inventory – a preliminary method of detecting depression in an outpatient setting.

Bilopancreatic diversion: surgery to reduce the size of the stomach and intestine to limit food intake and absorption.

Bolus rate: in terms of insulin pump therapy, this is the amount of insulin delivered for each meal or to correct a high blood glucose reading.

Bradycardia: rapid pulse.

Brittle Type 1 diabetes: where Type 1 diabetes is very difficult to control due to frequent and unexplained hypo- and hyperglycaemia.

Bulimia nervosa: a disorder characterised by binge eating, then vomiting or laxative abuse. Bupropion: an anti-depressant known to exacerbate the symptoms of psoriasis.

Calcific periarthritis: a condition where calcium deposits occur in the shoulder joints and soft tissues, restricting movement.

Cardiac tamponade: where the cardiac sac fills with blood, putting pressure on the heart.

Catabolism: chemical reactions that break down complex compounds with the release of energy.

Catecholamines: substances produced by the adrenal glands in response to stress, triggering the release of glucagon by the liver.

CBT: Cognitive Behavioural Therapy is a psychotherapeutic treatment addressing dysfunctional emotional patterns, maladaptive behaviours, and cognitive processes using goal-driven systematic methods.

Charcot joints: a chronic complication of diabetes where there is degeneration – predominantly of the foot joints – due to nerve damage, loss of sensation and excess areas of pressure.

Cheiroarthropathy: a disorder in which finger movement becomes limited as the hands become waxy and thickened.

Cholelithiasis: gallstones.

Chronic asthma: where the individual has a persistent wheeze and cough and is permanently breathless with frequent chest infections.

Chronic cortical hypofunction: an alternative name for Addison's disease.

Coeliac disease: a chronic autoimmune condition triggered by an intolerance to gluten (a protein found in cereal grains such as wheat) which cause chronic inflammation of the small bowel.

Cognition: the process of gaining knowledge, including perception, intuition and reasoning.

Cognitive reappraisal: when the individual is consciously aware of their cognitions and alters them accordingly.

Collagen: the most abundant protein in the body. It strengthens connective tissues and cushions the joints.

Colitis: a chronic condition where the colon and rectum become inflamed.

COM-B model: a theory of behaviour. COM-B posits behaviour as the result of an interaction between three components: capability, opportunity, and motivation (COM-B).

Comorbidities: the simultaneous presence of two or more diseases or medical conditions in a patient.

Common Sense model: used to understand people's responses to illness. The model proposes that illness perceptions directly influence coping strategies, which in turn influence outcomes.

Concordance: the extent to which an individual follows a given treatment regime.

Contraindications: drug interactions.

Control Theory: the idea that goal-setting and action planning can be used to change behaviour.

Cortisol: (Hydrocortisone) a glucocorticoid hormone which maintains the level of glucose in the blood plasma.

C-peptide: an essential but biologically inactive building block of insulin formed during the manufacture of insulin by the beta cells of the pancreas.

CSII: Continuous Subcutaneous Insulin Infusion.

DAFNE: Dosage Adjustment For Normal Eating.

Decisional balance. weighing up the pros and cons of changing health behaviour.

DESMOND: Diabetes Education and Self-Management for Ongoing and Newly Diagnosed.

Diabetes Insipidus: a rare condition affecting the pituitary gland, characterised by severe thirst and frequent urination that does not contain glucose.

Diabetic ketoacidosis (DKA): a medical emergency where there is severe disruption of the body's acidity balance due to prolonged hyperglycaemia.

Diabulimia: deliberate under-dosing or omission of insulin to achieve rapid weight loss by inducing hyperglycaemia and ketoacidosis. It is common in females with Type 1 diabetes.

Disordered eating: describes a range of eating-related problems, from dieting to anorexia and bulimia.

DKA: Diabetic Ketoacidosis – an acute and significant complication of Type 1 diabetes that occurs when blood glucose levels are consistently high (>15 mmol/L or >270 mg/dl) causing the breakdown of fats as an alternative source of energy to glucose that cannot be easily used in the lack of insulin.

Dyslipidaemia: a disorder of fat metabolism including lipoprotein under- or over-production, often manifesting as high blood cholesterol.

Dysthyroid optic neuropathy: a rare sight-threatening condition associated with Graves' disease (over-production of thyroid hormones) causing compression of the optic nerve.

Duodenum: the first part of the small intestine.

Eating disorders: psychological illnesses marked by disturbed eating behaviour, distorted food intake, disordered attitudes to eating, and inadequate methods of weight control.

ECT: electro-convulsive therapy.

Empowerment: increasing the individual's understanding of their diabetes and potential for self-care so that an informed choice can be made.

Exenatide: a blood glucose-lowering medication used to treat Type 2 diabetes, known to reduce itching in psoriasis.

Expressive repression: having awareness of cognitions and altering them accordingly.

External locus of control: a term describing individuals who do not feel as though they have any control over what happens to them because their lives are dictated by or subject to other people's actions.

Extrinsic asthma: where external factors (allergens) such as smoke, pollen, dust etc. trigger an attack.

Fluoxetine: an anti-depressant suitable for the treatment of depression in people with diabetes, but shown in some studies to exacerbate symptoms of psoriasis.

Folic acid: a water-soluble vitamin also known as vitamin B9.

FSH: Follicle Stimulating Hormone.

Gastroparesis: delayed stomach emptying causing bloating, early fullness and rarely, upper quadrant pain. The condition also occurs in people with diabetes due to autonomic nerve damage.

GI: Gastrointestinal.

Glucagon: attaches to the liver cells to make them release stored glucose quickly.

Glucocorticoid hormones: are mainly cortisol and adrenocortico-tropic hormone which are released during times of stress.

Glucocorticoid disruption: the release of hormones, such as cortisol, in times of stress.

Gluconeogenesis: the metabolic pathway resulting in the generation of glucose from non-carbohydrate sources, e.g. amino acids, glycerol or lactic acid enabling the release of glucose into the body.

Gluten: a protein found in cereal grains such as wheat, added to bread to make it rise.

Glycosylation: the breakdown of proteins into glucose.

GnTR: Gonadotrophin-releasing hormone.

Graves' disease: a condition describing the production of too much thyroxin by the thyroid gland.

Hashimoto's thyroiditis: also known as Chronic Lymphocytic Thyroiditis where autoimmune attack leads to too little thyroxin being produced.

HBM: Health Belief Model.

HbA1c (glycosylated haemoglobin): blood test measuring the amount of glucose sticking to the red blood cells over a three-month period.

HDL: High Density Lipids.

Hippocampus: the part of the brain responsible for consolidating memory.

Hyperglycaemia: high blood glucose levels >15.0 mmol/L.

Hyperleptinaemia: high levels of leptin, a hormone involved in reg-ulation of body fat, hunger and feeling full after meals.

Hyperlipidaemia: an increased level of harmful fats in the blood.

Hypertension: high blood pressure.

Hyperthyroidism: over-production of thyroid hormones.

Hypoglycaemia: low blood glucose levels <3.5 mmol/L.

Hypotension: low blood pressure.

Hypothalamus: a region of the brain situated below the thalamus, coordinating the autonomic nervous system and pituitary gland activity to regulate body temperature, hunger, thirst, sleep and emotional state.

Hypothalamic amenorrhea syndrome: absence of menstruation due to anorexia.

Hypothermia: a reduced body temperature below 35 degrees centigrade.

Hypothyroidism: under-production of thyroid hormones.

Immunosuppressant drugs: prevent organ rejection after transplant surgery by blocking immune system attack.

Incidence: the number of new cases of a disease that develop in a population.

Insula: part of the brain that is crucial to understanding what it feels like to be human. The starting place of social emotions such as guilt, atonement, moral intuition, empathy, and emotional response to music.

Insulin resistance: where the pancreas produces excess insulin to lower raised blood glucose levels in pre-diabetes or untreated Type 2 diabetes because the action of insulin on the cells is impaired by the presence of fat.

Interleukin-6: a substance associated with glucose intolerance that increases the inflammatory response of the immune system in severe illness.

Internal locus of control: a term describing an individual's perception of control over what happens to them because their decisions and actions are self-determined.

Internalising: having an internal rather than an external locus of control.

Intrinsic asthma: where there is no apparent external cause. Asthma can be episodic, where attacks occur at any time for a variable length and severity.

Iodide: iodine removed from the blood and combined with proteins in the thyroid gland to produce the hormone thyroxin.

Islet cell antibodies: proteins in the blood which destroy the insulin-producing beta cells of the pancreas.

Jejunum: the second part of the small intestine.

Lactate: a salt of lactic acid.

Lanugo: fine downy hair growth on the sides of the face and down the spine, associated with anorexia nervosa.

Lap band surgery: insertion of an adjustable gastric band.

Laparoscopic: gastric surgery performed via a small incision in the abdomen.

Laparoscopic sleeve gastrectomy: surgery to section off a small portion of the stomach so that it takes less food to become full.

Learned helplessness: a state where an individual feels they can do nothing about a situation and they become stressed, depressed, anxious and often hostile, losing their initiative as a result.

Leptin: a hormone made by fat cells that is involved in the regulation of body fat.

Leukopenia: anaemia and a low white blood cell count.

Liraglutide: a blood glucose-lowering medication used to treat Type 2 diabetes, known to reduce itching in psoriasis.

Lipolysis: regulation of protein synthesis and the mobilisation of fat controlled by growth hormone.

Lithium: an anti-depressant known to exacerbate the symptoms of psoriasis.

LH: Luteinising Hormone.

Macrophages: cells that remove bacteria and debris from the blood-stream and tissues.

Macrovascular: pertaining to the large blood vessels.

MBCT: Mindfulness-Based Cognitive Therapy.

MDI: multiple daily injections.

Metabolic syndrome: a group of pathophysiological states and cardiac risk factors which includes abdominal obesity, impaired glucose regulation, high blood fats, reduced high-density lipids, and hypertension. Insulin resistance means that glucose absorption in cells stimulated by insulin is reduced.

Microvascular: pertaining to the capillaries and small blood vessels.

Mixed hyperlipidaemia: a genetic, inherited disorder presenting as higher-than-normal levels of cholesterol, triglycerides, and other blood lipids. The disorder contributes to heart disease and early heart attacks.

Models: an example of patterns people may wish to follow.

MOI: Monoaminine Oxidase Inhibitor.

Morbidity: the state of being diseased – the morbidity rate being expressed as the number of cases of disease occurring within a particular number of the population.

Mortality: The number of deaths in a given period or from a given cause.

Motivation: in psychological terms, consisting of internal processes that spur us on to satisfy some need.

MDI: Multiple Daily Injections.

Myocardial infarction: destruction of a portion of the myocardium of the heart due to poor or absent blood supply.

Multimorbidities: defined as the coexistence of two or more chronic diseases; a common phenomenon, especially in older people.

Nephropathy: a chronic complication of diabetes caused by persistently high blood glucose levels leading to hardening of the kidney tissue and changes in the structure of the tubular epithelial cells.

Neurons: brain cells.

Neuropathy: a complex condition where nerve damage occurs, especially in the feet and hands.

Neuroplasticity: changing the way one thinks to enable the growth of new neuron connections in the brain.

Non-alcoholic fatty liver disease (NAFLD): a range of conditions caused by a build-up of fat in the liver; it is usually seen in people who are overweight or obese.

Normoglycaemia: a normal level of blood glucose within acceptable limits of 4.0–7.0 mmol/L.

Obesity: a body mass index of above 30 kg/m^2.

Obstructive sleep apnoea: OSA is a common condition where the walls of the throat relax and narrow during sleep, interrupting normal breathing. This may lead to regularly interrupted sleep, impacting on quality of life and increasing the risk of developing certain conditions.

Osteoarthritis: a very common condition due to wear and tear of the bones and joints (especially the weight-bearing knees and hips), also developing in bone following trauma.

Osteoarthropathy: a condition seen in people with Type 2 diabetes affecting the weight-bearing bones of the feet.

Osteopenia: a lack of bone density.

Osteoporosis: brittleness of the bones caused by lack of calcium.

Outcome expectancy: the expected results of diabetes self-management behaviour.

Orthostatic hypotension: low blood pressure.

Oxidative stress: cell breakdown where they die or are damaged beyond repair.

Peptides: small organic compounds made up of two or more amino acids.

Pericardial effusion: a collection of fluid in the pericardial sac surrounding the heart.

Peripheral neuropathy: a chronic complication of diabetes which occurs in two forms: diffuse neuropathy, commonly appearing as disorders of sensation in the extremities of the body; and distal polyneuropathy, affecting many nerves of the hands and feet.

Pessimistic attribution styles: consistently blaming oneself for negative things that happen and displaying passive (emotionally-focussed) rather than proactive coping strategies.

PET: Positron Emission Tomography.

Pneumothorax: air in the pleural space causing a lung to collapse.

Pneumoperineum: air in the abdominal cavity.

Polyautoimmunity: the presence of two or more autoimmune conditions, such as Type 1 diabetes and asthma, in the same individual.

Post-prandial: after meals.

Purging behaviour: classified as self-induced vomiting and laxative abuse which occurs at least twice a week for a period of three months.

Pre-diabetes: (also known as insulin resistance) where blood glucose levels are higher than normal but lower than established thresholds for diabetes itself.

Prevalence: refers to the pattern of occurrence of a disease.

Primary biliary cirrhosis: an autoimmune disease where there is slow, progressive destruction of the bile ducts causing bile and other toxins to build up in the liver, resulting in scarring and cirrhosis.

Primary sclerosing cholangitis: inflammation and obliterative fibrosis of the bile ducts inside and outside the liver, leading to liver failure and potentially bile duct and liver cancer.

Proactive consideration: when the individual considers the effect of a new behaviour.

Pro-insulin: the building blocks of insulin made by the beta cells of the pancreas.

Psoriasis: an autoimmune skin condition causing red, flaky, crusty patches covered with silvery scales appearing on the elbows, knees, scalp and lower back. These can become itchy and sore.

Pulmonary embolus: blockage of the pulmonary artery, or a branch of it, by a blood clot usually originating in the leg. Large pulmonary emboli can be fatal.

Reactive hypoglycaemia: a reduction in blood glucose level due to the body producing too much insulin.

Resistin: a substance released by the fat cells that 'resists' the action of insulin on the cells, preventing the lowering of blood glucose.

Retinopathy: a chronic complication of diabetes which describes a number of symptoms including abnormal dilation of the blood vessels of the eyes and haemorrhages of the retina. In advanced cases, the retina becomes heavily scarred and this may lead to blindness.

Self-efficacy: the individual's belief that they have the ability to achieve effective diabetes self-management.

Self-gratification: satisfaction.

Self-reactive influences: sensitivities.

Self-regulation theory: suggests that the individual reflects on their progress, feeding this information back to the health professionals providing their care, helping to maintain a behaviour change. However, this reflection on the need to achieve an improvement may become demotivating.

Severe hypoglycaemia: disabling low blood glucose levels requiring the assistance of another person.

Serotonin: a hormone that gives us a sense of wellbeing. It acts as a neurotransmitter to relay signals from one area of the brain to another.

Sickness behaviour: a coordinated set of behaviour changes that develop in all cases of illness that includes low motivation to eat, listlessness, fatigue, malaise, a reduced interest in social activity, change in sleep patterns, inability to experience pleasure, an exaggerated response to pain and lack of concentration.

Sleep apnoea: where fat around the neck impedes breathing during sleep.

SMAS: Super Mesenteric Artery Syndrome, where the duodenum is compressed between the spine and the aorta.

SNRIs: Selective Noradrenaline Reuptake Inhibitors – an antidepressant medication.

SOC: Stages of Change model.

Sorbitol: a substance metabolised from excessive glucose which triggers chronic diabetes complications as the large sorbitol molecules damages cells.

SSRIs: Selective Serotonin Reuptake Inhibitors – an anti-depressant medication.

Status asthmaticus: where an asthma attack is severe and lasts for more than 24 hours with no response to medication, leading to increased heart rate and potential loss of conciseness.

Steatohepatitis: fatty liver disease.

Steatosis: increased liver enzymes associated with intravenous feeding of dextrose to patients with anorexia.

Stricture: the growth of scar tissue following surgery or injury resulting in narrowing, e.g. intestinal stricture following bariatric surgery.

Systemic conditions: having an effect on the whole body (such as diabetes).

Tension pneumothorax: where a valve develops in the lung allowing air to enter into the pleural space which cannot escape, pushing the heart, lungs, trachea, oesophagus and other structures towards the unaffected lung.

TCA: tricyclic anti-depressants.

T-cells: thymus lymphocytes circulating in the blood and lymphatic fluid that trigger the immune system to fight infection.

Thalamus: the relay station of the brain.

The hygiene hypothesis: proposes that infections in early childhood may reduce the risk of allergic diseases by strengthening the immune system's defence.

Thrombopenia: a low red blood cell count.

TRA: Theory of Reasoned Action.

TSH: Thyroid Stimulating Hormone.

Thyrotoxicosis: over-production of thyroid hormones by the thyroid gland itself, or due to ineffective storage or leakage of the hormones.

Transaminases: enzymes produced by the liver which break down amino acids and convert them to energy storage molecules.

TSH: Thyroid Stimulating Hormone.

Vasoconstriction of the arteries: narrowing.

Vasodilation of the arteries: widening.

Wernick'e encephalopathy: a neurological disorder caused by vitamin B1 (thiamine) deficiency.

References

Abdullah, A., Stoelwidner, J., Shortreed, S. (2011) The duration of obesity and the risk of developing Type 2 diabetes. *Public Health Nutrition* 14(1): 119–126.

Abella, E., Feliu, E., Granada, I. (2002) Bone marrow changes in anorexia nervosa are correlated with the amount of weight loss and not with other clinical findings. *American Journal of Clinical Pathology* 118: 582–588.

Abid, N., Mcglone, O., Cardwell, C., et al. (2011) Clinical and metabolic effects of gluten free diet in children with Type 1 diabetes and coeliac disease. *Pediatric Diabetes* 12(4): part 1, 322–325.

Abiles, V., Rodríguez-Ruiz, S., Abiles, J., et al. (2010) Psychological characteristics of morbidly obese candidates for bariatric surgery. *Obesity Surgery* 20(2): 161–167.

Abramson, J., Berger, A., Krumholz, H.M., et al. (2001) Depression and risk of heart failure among older persons with isolated systolic hypertension. *Archive of Internal Medicine* 161(14): 1725–1730.

Ackard, D.M., Neumark-Sztainer, V.N., Schmitz, K.H., et al. (2008) Disordered eating and body dissatisfaction in adolescents with Type 1 diabetes and a population-based comparison sample: comparative prevalence and clinical implications. *Pediatric Diabetes* 9: 312–319.

Adams, T.D., Gress, R.E., Smith, S.C., et al. (2007) Long-term mortality after gastric bypass surgery. *New England Journal of Medicine* 357: 753–761.

Aggarwal, S., Lebwohl, B., Green, P.H.R. (2012) Screening for celiac disease in average-risk and high-risk populations. *Therapeutic Advances in Gastroenterology* 5(1): 37–47.

Ahmad, L.A., Crandall, J.P. (2010) Type 2 diabetes prevention: a review. *Clinical Diabetes* 28(2): 53–58.

Aikens, J.E. (2010) Prospective associations between emotional distress and poor outcomes in Type 2 diabetes. *Diabetes Care* 35: 2472–2478.

Al-Abadie, M.S., Kent, G.G., Gawkrodger, D.J. (1994) The relationship between stress and the onset and exacerbation of psoriasis and other skin conditions. *British Journal of Dermatology* 130: 199–203.

Al-Arouj, A., Khalil, A., Buse, J., et al. (2010) Recommendations for management of diabetes during Ramadan. *Diabetes Care* 33(10): 1895–1904.

Alberti, G. (2002) The DAWN (Diabetes Attitudes, Wishes, and Needs) study. *Practical Diabetes International* 19: 22–24.

Algoblan, A., Alalfi, M., Khan, M. (2014) Mechanism linking diabetes mellitus and obesity. *DMSO.* 7: 587–591.

Aliyu, I. (2014) Acute psychosis following diabetic ketoacidosis in an 11-year-old: management challenges in a resource-limited setting. *Sudan Medical Monitor* 9(2). http://www.sudanmedicalmonitor.org

Aljahlan, M., Lee, K.C., Toth, E. (1999) Limited joint mobility in diabetes. *Postgraduate Medicine* 105(2): 99–106.

Alpsoy, E., Ozcan, E., Cetin, L., et al. (1998) Is the efficacy of topical corticosteroid therapy for psoriasis vulgaris enhanced by concurrent moclobemide therapy? A double-blind, placebo-controlled study. *Journal of the American Academic Dermatology* 38: 197–200.

American Diabetes Association (2020) Comprehensive Medical Evaluation and Assessment of Comorbidities: Standards of Medical Care in Diabetes-2020. *Diabetes Care* 43(Supplement 1): S37–S47. doi:10.2337/dc20-S004

American Diabetes Association (2012) Diagnosis and classification of diabetes mellitus. *Diabetes Care* 35: S64–S71.

American Diabetes Association (2003) Treatment of hypertension in adults with diabetes. *Diabetes Care* 26(1): S80–S82.

American Psychiatric Association (2013) *Diagnostic Statistical Manual of Mental Disorders.* 5th edition, Washington DC: American Psychiatric Association.

American Psychiatric Association (2006) *Practice Guideline for the Treatment of Patients with Eating Disorders.* 3rd edition. http://www.psych.org/psych_pract

Anderbro, T., Amsberg, S., Moberg, E., et al. (2010) Fear of hypoglycaemia in adults with Type 1 diabetes. *Diabetic Medicine* 27(10): 1151–1158.

Anderson, R. J., Freedland, K. E., Clouse, R. E., et al. (2001) The prevalence of comorbid depression in adults with diabetes: A meta-analysis. *Diabetes Care* 24(6), 1069–1078.

Arkkila, P.E., Kantola, I.M., Vikkari, J.S. (1997) Limited joint mobility in non-insulin-dependent diabetic patients: correlation to control of diabetes, atherosclerotic vascular disease, and other diabetic complications. *Journal of Diabetes Complications* 11(4): 208–217.

Arkkila, P.E., Kantola, I.M., Vikkari, J.S. (1994) Limited joint movement in Type 1 diabetic patients: correlation to other complications. *Journal of Internal Medicine* 236(2): 215–216.

Aronson, D. (2008) Hyperglycemia and the pathobiology of diabetic complications. *Advanced Cardiology* 45: 1–16.

Arora, M., Barquera, S., Farpour-Lambert, N.J., et al. (2019) Stigma and obesity: the crux of the matter. *The Lancet.* https://www.thelancet.com/journals/lanpub/article/PIIS2468-2667(19)30186-0/fulltext

Asimakopoulou, K.G., Fox, C., Spimpolo, J., et al. (2008) The impact of different time frames of risk communication on Type 2 diabetes patients' understanding and memory for risk of coronary heart disease and stroke. *Diabetic Medicine* 25(7): 811–817.

Aspinwall, L.G., Tedeschi, R. (2010) The value of positive psychology for health psychology: progress and pitfalls in examining the relationship of positive phenomenon to health. *Annals of Behavioural Medicine* 39(1): 4–15.

Asvoid, B.O., Sandt, T., Hestad, K., et al. (2010) Cognitive function in Type 1 diabetes with early exposure to severe hypoglycaemia. *Diabetes Care* 33: 1945–1947.

Auer, R.N. (2004) Hypoglycaemic brain damage. *Metabolic Brain Disease* 19: 169–175.

Azizi, F. (2002) Research in Islamic fasting and health. *Annuls of Saudi Medicine* 22:186–191.

Bächle, C., Stahl-Pehe, A., Rosenbauer, J. (2016) Disordered eating and insulin restriction in youths receiving intensified insulin treatment: Results from a nationwide population-based study. *International Journal of Eating Disorders* 49(2): 191–196.

Badescu, S.V., Tataru, C., Koylinska, L., et al. (2016) The association between diabetes mellitus and depression. *Journal of Medicine and Life* 9(20): 120–125.

Baker, R.A., Pikalov, A., Tran, Q.V., et al. (2009) Atypical antipsychotic drugs and diabetes mellitus in the US Food and Drug Administration Adverse Event database: A systematic Bayesian signal detection analysis. *Psychopharmacology Bulletin* 42: 11–31.

Bakker, S.F., Tushuizen, M.E., Stokvis-Brantsma, W.H.S., et al. (2013a) Frequent delay of coeliac disease diagnosis in symptomatic patients with Type 1 diabetes mellitus: clinical and genetic characteristics. *European Journal of Internal Medicine* 24(5): 456–460.

Bakker, S.F., Tushuizen, M.E., von Blomberg, M.E., et al. (2013b) Type 1 diabetes and celiac disease in adults: glycemic control and diabetic complications. *Acta Diabetologica*, 50(3): 319–324.

Balci, A., Balci, D.D., Yonden, Z., et al. (2010) Increased amount of visceral fat in patients with psoriasis contributes to metabolic syndrome. *Dermatology* 220: 32–37.

Balkau, B., Vol, S., Loko, S., et al. (2010) Epidemiologic study on the Insulin Resistance Syndrome Study Group. High baseline insulin levels associated with 6-year incident observed sleep apnoea. *Diabetes Care* 33: 1044–1049.

Bandura, A. (2001) Social cognitive theory: an agentic perspective. *Annual Review of Psychology* 52: 1–26.

Bandura, A. (2000) Health promotion from the perspective of social cognitive theory. In: Norman, P., Abraham, C., Conner, M. (Eds) *Understanding and Changing Health Behaviour: From Health Beliefs to Self-Regulation.* Harwood Academic: Amsterdam.

Bandura, A. (1991) Social cognitive theory of self-regulation. *Theories of Cognitive Self-Regulation* 50: 248–287.

Barlow, S.E. (2007) Expert committee recommendations regarding the prevention, assessment and treatment of child and adolescent overweight and obesity: summary report. *Pediatrics* 120: S164–S192.

Basavaraj, K.H., Ashok, N.M., Rashmi, R., et al. (2010) The role of drugs in the induction and/or exacerbation of psoriasis. *International Journal of Dermatology* 49: 1351–1361.

Baumeister, R.F., Tierney, J. (2012) *Willpower: Rediscovering the Greatest Human Strength*. USA: Random House, Penguin Press.

Baumeister, R.F. (2003) Ego depletion and self-regulation failure: a resource model of self-control. *Alcohol Clinical Expertise and Research* 27: 281–284.

BBC (8th October, 2020) Coronavirus: Year-long waits for NHS care at highest since 2008. https://www.bbc.co.uk/news/health-54463441

Becker, M.H., Janz, N.K. (1985) The health belief model applied to understanding diabetes regime compliance. *The Diabetes Educator* 11: 41–47.

Beer, S.F., Parr, J.H., Temple, R.C., et al. (1989) The effect of thyroid disease on proinsulin and C-peptide levels. *Clinical Endocrinology* 30(4): 379–383.

Bener, A, Ghuloum, S., Al-Hamaq, A.O., et al. (2012) Association between psychological distress and gastrointestinal symptoms in diabetes mellitus. *World Journal of Diabetes*3: 123–129.

Benchimol, E.I., Manuel, D.G., To, T., et al. (2015) Asthma, Type 1 and Type 2 diabetes mellitus and inflammatory bowel disease among South Asian immigrants to Canada and their children: a population-based cohort study. *PLoS One* 10(4): e0123599.

Berger, J.R. (2004) The neurological complications of bariatric surgery. *Archive of Neurology* 61: 1185–1189.

Bermudez, O., Sommer, J. (2012) Beyond "diabulimia": the dual diagnosis of eating disorder and diabetes. *The Pulse* 31(2): 9–12.

Berry, J. (2016) Does health literacy matter? NHS England. https://www.england.nhs.uk/blog/jonathan-berry/

Betterle, C., Lazzaratto, F., Spadaccino, A.C., et al. (2006) Celiac disease in North Italian patients with autoimmune Addison's disease. *European Journal of Endocrinology*, 154(2): 275–279.

Betterle, C., Dal Pra C., Mantero, F., et al. (2002) Autoimmune adrenal insufficiency and autoimmune polyendocrine syndromes: autoantibodies, autoantigens and their application in diagnosis and disease prediction. *Endocrine Review* 23: 327–364.

Betterle, C., Volpato, M., Greggio, A.N. (1996) Type 2 polyglandular autoimmune disease (Schmidt's syndrome). *Journal of Pediatric Endocrinology and Metabolism* 9:113–123.

Biagi, F., Campanella, J., Soriani, A., et al. (2006) Prevalence of coeliac disease in Italian patients affected by Addison's disease. *Scandinavian Journal of Gastroenterology* 41(3): 302–305.

Black, M.H., Anderson, A., Bell, R.A., et al. (2011) Prevalence of asthma and its association with glycemic control among youth with diabetes. *Pediatrics* 128: e839–e847.

Biddle, S.J., Fox, K.R., Boutcher, S.H. (Eds.) (2000) *Physical Activity and Psychological Well-Being*. New York: Routledge.

Biffl, W.L., Narayanan, V., Gaudiani, J.L., et al. (2010) The management of pneumothorax in patients with anorexia nervosa: A case report and review of the literature. *Patient Safety in Surgery* 4: 1.

Bishop, G.D., Smelser, N.J., Baltes, P.B. (2001) *Emotions and Health*. Oxford: Pergamon.

Bluestone, J.A., Buckner, J.H., Fitch, M., et al. (2015) Type 1 diabetes immunotherapy using polyclonal regulatory T cells. *Science Translational Medicine* 7(315): 315ra189.

Bocchieri, L.E., Meana, M., Fisher, B.L. (2002) A review of psychosocial outcomes of surgery for morbid obesity. *Journal of Psychosomatic Research* 52(3): 155–165.

Boden, G., Sargrad, K., Homko, C., et al. (2005) Effect of a low-carbohydrate diet on appetite, blood glucose levels and insulin resistance in obese patients with Type 2 diabetes. *Annals of Internal Medicine* 142: 403–411.

Boden, G., Hoeldtke, R.D. (2003) Nerves, fat, and insulin resistance. *New England Journal of Medicine* 349: 1966–1967.

Boehncke, W., Boehncke, S., Tobin, A.M. (2011) The 'psoriatic march': a concept of how severe psoriasis may drive cardiovascular comorbidity. *Experimental Dermatology* 20: 303–307.

Boehncke, W.H., Boehncke, S., Buerger, C. (2012) Beyond immunopathogenesis. Insulin resistance and "epidermal dysfunction". *Der Hautarzt* 63: 178–183.

Boule, N.G., Haddad, E., Kenny, G.P., et al. (2001) Effects of exercise on glycemic control and body mass in Type 2 diabetes mellitus: a meta-analysis of controlled clinical trials. *Journal of the American Medical Association* 286 (10): 1218–1227.

Brauchli, Y.B., Jick, S.S., Meier, C.R. (2008) Psoriasis and the risk of incident diabetes mellitus: a population-based study. *British Journal of Dermatology* 159:1331–1337.

Bradley, M.M., Lang, P.J. (2000) Measuring emotion: Behavior, feeling, and physiology. In: Nadel, R.D.L.L. (Ed.) *Cognitive Neuroscience of Emotion*. New York: Oxford University Press.

Bradshaw, B.G., Richardson, G.E., Kulkarni, K. (2007a) Thriving with diabetes: an introduction to the resiliency approach for diabetes educators. *Diabetes Educator* 33: 643–649.

Bradshaw, B.G., Richardson, G.E., Kumpfer, K., et al. (2007b) Determining the efficacy of a resiliency training approach in adults with Type 2 diabetes. *Diabetes Educator* 33: 650–659.

Bremmer, S., Van Voorhees, A.S., Hsu, S., et al. (2010) Obesity and psoriasis: from the Medical Board of the National Psoriasis Foundation. *Journal of the American Academy of Dermatology* 63: 1058–1069.

Broadbent, E., Schoones, J. W., Tiemensma, J., et al. (2019). A systematic review of patients' drawing of illness: Implications for research using the common sense model. *Health Psychology Review*. doi: 10.1080/17437199.2018.1558088

Broome, A., Llewelyn, S. (1995) *Health Psychology: Process and Application*. London: Chapman and Hall.

Brown, L.C., Newman, S.C., Majumdar, S.R., et al. (2005) Depression increased risk of Type 2 diabetes in young adults. *Diabetes Care* 28: 1063–1067.

Brown, R.F., Bartrop, R., Beaumont, P., et al. (2005) Bacterial infections in anorexia nervosa: delayed recognition increases complications. *International Journal of Eating Disorders* 37: 261–265.

Brown, S.A., Sharpless, S.L. (2004) Osteoporosis: An under-appreciated complication of diabetes. *Clinical Diabetes* 22(1): 10–21.

Brown, A.F., Mangione, C.M., Saliba, D., et al. (2003) Guidelines for improving the care of the older person with diabetes mellitus. *Journal of American Geriatric Society* 51: S265–S280.

Buchwald, H., Estok, R., Fahrbach, K., et al. (2009) Weight and Type 2 diabetes after bariatric surgery: systematic review and meta-analysis. *American Journal of Medicine* 122: 248–256, e5.

Buchwald, H. (2005) Health implications of bariatric surgery. *Journal of the American College of Surgery* 200: 593–604.

Buchwald, H., Avidor, Y., Brau, E., et al. (2004) Bariatric surgery: a systematic review and meta-analysis. *Journal of the American Medical Association* 292(14): 1724–1737.

Bulik, C.M., Hoffman, E.R., Von Holle, R. (2010) Unplanned pregnancy in women with anorexia nervosa. *Obstetrics & Gynaecology* 116: 1136–1140.

Bulik, C.M., Sullivan, P.F., Fear, J.L. (1999) Fertility and reproduction in women with anorexia nervosa: a controlled study. *Journal of Clinical Psychiatry* 60:130–135.

Burns, R.B. (2001) *Essential Psychology*, Second edition. Dordrecht, The Netherlands: Kluwer Academic Publishers.

Camarca, M.E., Mozzillo, E., Nugnes, R., et al. (2012) Celiac disease in Type 1 diabetes mellitus. *Italian Journal of Pediatrics* 38, article 10.

Cameron, L., Leventhal, H. (2002) *The Self-Regulation of Health and Illness Behaviour.* Routledge.

Carney, R.M., Freedland, K.E. (2003) Depression, mortality, and medical morbidity in patients with coronary heart disease. *Biological Psychiatry* 54: 241–247.

Carthenon, M.R., Kinder, L.S., Fair, J.M., et al. (2003) Symptoms of depression as a risk factor for incident diabetes: findings from the National Health and Nutrition Examination Epidemiologic Follow-up Study, 1971-1992. *American Journal of Epidemiology* 158(5): 416–423.

Cataldo, F., Marino, V. (2003) Increased prevalence of autoimmune diseases in first-degree relatives of patients with celiac disease. *Journal of Pediatric Gastroenterology and Nutrition* 36 (4): 470–473.

Center for Disease Control and Prevention (2011) *National Diabetes Factsheet.* Atlanta, Georgia: Centre for Disease Control and Prevention.

Cerutti, F., Bruno, G., Chiarelli, F., et al. (2004) Younger age at onset and sex predict celiac disease in children and adolescents with Type 1 diabetes: an Italian multicenter study. *Diabetes Care* 27(6): 1294–1298.

Cettour-Rose, P., Theander-Carrillo, C., Asensio, C., et al. (2005) Hypothyroidism in rats decreases peripheral glucose utilisation, a defect partially corrected by central leptin infusion. *Diabetologia* 48(4): 624–633.

Chan, R., Brooks, R., Erlich, J., et al. (2009) The effects of kidney-disease-related loss on long-term dialysis patients' depression and quality of life: positive affect as a mediator. *Clinical Journal of the American Society of Nephrology* 4: 160–167.

Ch'ng, C.L., Jones, M.K., Kingham, J.G.C. (2007) Celiac disease and autoimmune thyroid disease. *Clinical Medicine and Research* 5(3): 184–192.

Chanoine, J.P., Hampl, S., Jensen, C., et al. (2005) Effect of Orlistat on weight and body composition in obese adolescents: a randomized controlled trial. *Journal of the American Medical Association* 293(23): 2873–2883.

Chapman, D.P., Perry, G.S., Strine, T.W. (2005) The vital link between chronic disease and depressive disorders. *Preventing Chronic Disease* 2(1): A14. http://www.cdc.gov/pcd/issues/2005/

Chen, H.S., Wu, T.E.J., Jap, T.S., et al. (2007) Subclinical hypothyroidism is a risk factor for nephropathy and cardiovascular diseases in Type 2 diabetic patients. *Diabetic Medicine* 24(12): 1336–1344.

Chew, B-H., Shariff-Ghazali, S., Fernandez, A. (2014) Psychological aspects of diabetes care: effecting behavioural change in patients. *Diabetes Care* 5(6): 796–808.

Chiba, M., Suzuki, S., Hinokio, Y., et al. (2000) Tyrosine hydroxylase gene microsatellite polymorphism associated with insulin resistance in depressive disorder. *Metabolism* 49:1145–1149.

Clark, M.L., Utz, S.W. (2014) Social determinants of Type 2 diabetes and health in the United States. *World Journal of Diabetes* 5: 296–304.

Clark, M. (2004a) *Understanding Diabetes*. West Sussex, England: John Wiley & Sons Ltd.

Clark, M. (2004b) Identification and treatment of depression in people with diabetes. *Diabetes and Primary Care* 5(3): 124–127.

Clarke, C.F., Piesowicz, A.T., Spathis, G.S. (1990) Limited joint mobility in children and adolescents with Type 1 diabetes mellitus. *Annals of Rheumatic Disease* 49(4): 236–237.

Ciechanowski, P.S., Katon, W.J., Russo, J.E., et al. (2003) The relationship of depressive symptoms to symptom reporting, self-care, and glucose control in diabetes. *General Hospital Psychiatry* 25: 246–252.

Ciechanowski, P.S., Katon, W.J., Russo, J.E., et al. (2001) The patient-provider relationship: attachment theory and adherence to treatment in diabetes. *General Hospital Psychiatry* 158(1): 29–35.

Ciechanowski, P.S., Katon, W.J., Russo, J.E. (2000) Depression and diabetes: impact of depressive symptoms on adherence, function, and costs. *Archive of Internal Medicine* 160: 3278–3285.

Coates, P.S., Fernstrom, J.D., Fernstrom, M.H., et al. (2004) Gastric bypass surgery for morbid obesity leads to an increase in bone turnover and a decrease in bone mass. *Journal of Clinical Endocrinology and Metabolism* 89: 1061–1065.

Cohen, A.D., Gilutz, H., Henkin, Y., et al. (2007) Psoriasis and the metabolic syndrome. *Acta Dermatology and Venereology* 87: 506–509.

Cohen, S.T., Welch, G., Jacobson, A.M., et al. (1997) The association of lifetime psychiatric illness and increased retinopathy in patients with Type I diabetes mellitus. *Psychosomatics* 38(2):98–108.

Coimbra, S., Oliveira, H., Reis, F., et al. (2010) Circulating adipokine levels in Portuguese patients with psoriasis vulgaris according to body mass index, severity and therapy. *Journal of European Academic Dermatology and Venereology* 24: 1386–1394.

Colton, P.A., Olmsted, M.P., Daneman, D., et al. (2007) Five-year prevalence & persistence of disturbed eating behaviour and eating disorders in girls with Type 1 diabetes. *Diabetes Care* 30: 2861–2862.

Colton, P.A., Olmsted, M.P., Daneman, D., et al. (2004) Disturbed eating disorders in pre-teen & early teenage girls with Type 1 diabetes: a case-controlled study. *Diabetes Care* 27: 1654–1659.

Connor, M., Norman, P. (2015) *Predicting Health Behaviour: Research and Practice with Social Practice.* Buckingham: Open University Press.

Cox, N.H., Gordon, P.M., Dodd, H. (2002) Generalized pustule aranderythrodermic psoriasis associated with Bupropion treatment. *British Journal of Dermatology* 146:1061–1063.

Cranston, I. (2005) *Diabetes and the Brain.* In: Diabetes: Chronic Complications, Shaw, K.M. & Cummings, M.H. (Eds.), second edition. Chichester, West Sussex: John Wiley & Sons Limited.

Criego, A., Scott, M.S., Crow, M.D., et al. (2009) Eating Disorders and Diabetes: Screening and Detection. *Diabetes Spectrum* 22(3): 143–146.

Crookes, P.F. (2006) Surgical treatment of morbid obesity. *Annual Review of Medicine* 57: 243–264.

Crow, S.J., Keel, P.K., Kendall, D. (2000) Relationship of weight and eating disorders in Type 2 diabetic patients: A multicentre study. *International Journal of Eating Disorders* 28: 68–77.

Dae-Jin, K., Yu, J.H., Mi-Seon, S., et al. (2016) Hyperglycaemia reduces efficiency of brain networks in subjects with Type 2 diabetes. *Plos One* https://journals.plos.org/plosone/article?id=10.1371/journal.pone.0157268

Dalle-Grave, R., Calugi, S., Marchesini, G. (2008) Is amenorrhea a useful criterion for the diagnosis of anorexia nervosa? *Behaviour Research Therapy* 46: 1290–1296.

Dalsgaard, E.M., Vestergaard, M., Skriver, M.V., et al. (2014) Psychological distress, cardiovascular complications and mortality among people with screen-detected Type 2 diabetes: follow-up of the ADDITION-Denmark trial. *Diabetologia* 57: 710–717.

Daneman, D., Rodin, G., Jones, J., et al. (2002) Eating disorders in adolescent girls and young women with Type 1 diabetes. *Diabetes Spectrum* 15(2): 83–105.

Dantzer, R. (2004) Cytokine-induced sickness behaviour: a neuroimmune response to activation of innate immunity. *European Journal of Pharmacology* 500: 399–411.

Dantzer, R. (2001) Cytokine-induced sickness behavior: where do we stand? *Brain Behaviour and Immunity* 15: 7–24.

Dario Health (2019) *Techniques for Successful Diabetes Management.* Dario Health, Kindle Edition.

Davidson, K., Jonahs, B.S., Dixon, K.E., et al. (2000) Do depression symptoms predict early hypertension incidence in young adults in the CARDIA study? Coronary Artery Risk Development in Young Adults. *Archive of Internal Medicine* 160(10): 1495–1500.

Day, J.L. (1995) Why should patients do what we ask them to do? *Patient Education and Counselling* 26 (1–3): 113–118.

De Boer, I.H., Bangalore, S., Benetos, A., et al. (2017) Diabetes and Hypertension: A Position Statement by the American Diabetes Association. *Diabetes Care* 40(9):1273–1284. doi:10.2337/dci17-0026

De Caprio, C., Alfano, A., Senatore, I. (2006) Severe acute liver damage in anorexia nervosa: two case reports *Nutrition* 22; 572–575.

De Groot, M., Anderson, R., Freedland, K.E., et al. (2001) Association of depression and diabetes complications: a meta-analysis. *Psychosomatic Medicine* 63: 619–630.

Den Hollander, J.G., Wulkan, R.W., Mantel, M.J., et al. (2005) Correlation between severity of thyroid dysfunction and renal function. *Clinical Endocrinology* 62(4): 423–427.

Department of Health (2003) *National Service Framework for Diabetes: Standards Document.* London: Department of Health.

Department of Health (2002) *Priorities for the Diabetes National Service Framework (NSF) for England and Wales.* www.doh.gov.uk/nsf/diabetes

Department of Health (2001) *National Service Framework for Diabetes.* Bit.ly/ DHNSFDiabetes

Dew, M.A. (1998) *Psychiatric Disorder in the Context of Physical Illness. Adversity, Stress, and Psychopathology.* New York: Oxford University Press.

de Zwaan, M., Hilbert, A., Swan-Kremeier, L., et al. (2010) Comprehensive interview assessment of eating behavior 18–35 months after gastric bypass surgery for morbid obesity. *Surgery for Obesity and Related Diseases* 6(1): 79–85.

Dharmalingam, M., Yamasandhi, P. (2018) Non-alcoholic fatty liver disease and Type 2 diabetes mellitus. *Indian Journal Endocrinology and Metabolism* 22(3): 421-428. doi:10.4103/ijem.IJEM_585_17

Diabetes Control and Complications Trial Research Group (1993) The effect of intensified treatment on the development and progression of long-term complications of insulin dependent diabetes mellitus. *New England Journal of Medicine* 329: 977–986.

Diabetes.co.uk (2019a) Prevalence of diabetes. https://www.diabetes.co.uk/diabetes-prevalence.html#:~:text=It%20is%20estimated%20that%20415,with%20diabetes%20worldwide%20by%202040

Diabetes UK (2019b) *Diabetes and Emotional Health – A Practical Guide for Healthcare Professionals Supporting Adults with Type 1 and Type 2 Diabetes.* London: Diabetes UK, 2nd Edition. https://www.diabetes.org.uk/professionals/resources/shared-practice/psychological-care/emotional-health-professionals-guide

Diabetes UK (2018) Diabetes and diabulimia. https://www.diabetes.org.uk/guide-to-diabetes/life-with-diabetes/diabulimia

Diabetes UK (2017) The Future of Diabetes Report. https://www.diabetes. org.uk/ resources-s3/2017-11/1111B%20The%20future%20of%20diabetes%20report_FINAL_.pdf

Diabetes UK (2016) Diabetes and mental health. https://www.diabetes.org.uk/ resources-s3/2018-08/Diabetes%20and%20Mental%20Health%20%28PDF%2C%205.7MB%29.pdf

Diabetes UK (2008) *Early Identification of Type 2 Diabetes and the new Vascular Risk Assessment and Management Programme.* Position Statement Update. London: Diabetes UK.

Diabetes UK (2000) *What Diabetes Care to Expect*. London: Diabetes UK.

DiMatteo, M.R., Lepper, H.S., Croghan, T.W. (2000) Depression is a risk factor for non-compliance with medical treatment: meta-analysis of the effects of anxiety and depression on patient adherence. *Archive of Internal Medicine* 160: 2101–2107.

Dimitriadis, G., Mitrou, P., Lambadiari, V., et al. (2006) Insulin action in adipose tissue and muscle in hypothyroidism. *Journal of Clinical Endocrinology and Metabolism* 91(12): 4930–4937.

Dixon, A. (2008) *Motivation and Confidence: What Does it Take to Change Behaviour?* The Kings Fund: London, England.

Donkin, L., Ellis, C.J., Powell, R., et al. (2006) Illness perceptions predict reassurance following a negative exercise stress testing result. *Psychology and Health* 21: 421–430.

Donnovan, P.T., MacDonald, T.M., Morris, A.D. (2002) Adherence to prescribed oral hypoglycaemic medications in a population of patients with Type 2 diabetes: a retrospective cohort study. *Diabetic Medicine* 19: 274–284.

Docx, M.K., Gewillig, M., Simons, A., et al. (2010) Pericardial effusions in adolescent girls with anorexia nervosa: clinical course and risk factors. *Eating Disorders* 18: 218–225.

Drucker, D.J., Sherman, S.I., Gorelick, F.S. (2010) Incretin-based therapies for the treatment of Type 2 diabetes: evaluation of the risks and benefits. *Diabetes Care* 33: 428–433.

Druss, B.G., Rohrbaugh, R.M., Rosenheck, R.A. (2000) Depressive symptoms and health costs in older medical patients. *General Hospital Psychiatry* 156(3):477–479.

Ducat, L., Phillipson, L.H., Anderson, B. (2014) The mental health comorbidities of diabetes. *Journal of the American Medical Association* https://jamanetwork.com/journals/jama/article-abstract/1888681

Duckworth, A.L. (2011) The significance of self-control. *Proceedings of the National Academy of Science* 108: 2639–2640.

Dymek, M.P., le Grange, D., Neven, K., et al. (2001) Quality of life and psychosocial adjustment in patients after Roux-en-Y Gastric Bypass: a brief report. *Obesity Surgery* 11(1): 32–39.

Dyson, P. (2012) Dietary interventions and weight reduction in people with Type 2 diabetes. Primary Care Diabetes Society. https://www.pcdsociety.org/resources/details/dietary-interventions-and-weight-reduction-in-people-with-type-2diabetes#:~:text=Studies%20investigating%20the%20effect%20of,replacements%20and%20commercial%20diet%20groups.

Eder, K., Baffy, N., Falus, A., Fulop, A.K. (2009) The major inflammatory mediator interleukin-6 and obesity. *Inflammation. Research* 58: 727–736.

Edgar, K. A., Skinner, T. C. (2003) Illness representations and coping as predictors of emotional well-being in adolescents with Type 1 diabetes. *Journal of Pediatric Psychology* 28(7): 485–493.

Egede, L.E., Zheng, D., Simpson, K. (2002) Comorbid depression is associated with increased health care use and expenditures in individuals with diabetes. *Diabetes Care* 25(3): 464–470.

Ehrlich, S., Burghardt, R., Weiss, D., et al. (2008) Glial and neuronal damage markers in patients with anorexia nervosa. *Journal of Neuralogical Transmission* 115: 921–927.

Elfstrom, P., Montgomery, S.M., Kampe, O., et al. (2008) Risk of thyroid disease in individuals with celiac disease. *The Journal of Clinical Endocrinology and Metabolism* 93(10): 3915–3921.

Elfstrom, P., Montgomery, S.M., Kampe, O., et al. (2007) Risk of primary adrenal insufficiency in patients with celiac disease. *The Journal of Clinical Endocrinology and Metabolism* 92(9): 3595–3598.

Erdogan, M., Canataraglu, A., Ganidaqil, S., et al. (2011) Metabolic syndrome prevalence in subclinic and overt hypothyroid patients and the relation among metabolic syndrome parameters. *Journal of Endocrinological Investigation* 34(7): 488–492.

Erickson, S.J., Robinson, T.N., Farish-Haydel, K., et al. (2000) Are overweight children unhappy? Body mass index, depressive symptoms, and overweight concerns in elementary school children. *Archives of Pediatrics & Adolescent Medicine* 154(9): 931–935.

Estour, B., Germain, N., Diconne, E. (2010) Hormonal profile heterogeneity and short-term physical risk in restrictive anorexia nervosa. *Journal of Clinical Endocrinology and Metabolism*. 95: 2203–2210.

Fadhil, A., Wang, Y. (2019) Health behaviour change techniques in diabetes management applications: a systematic review. *Medicine Plus* https://arxiv.org/ftp/arxiv/papers/1904/1904.09884.pdf

Fazeli, P.K., Klibanski, A. (2014) Bone metabolism in anorexia nervosa. *Current Osteoporosis Report* 12: 82–89.

Felig, P. (1979) Starvation. In: *Endocrinology*. DeGroot, L.J. (Ed.) New York: Grune & Stratton.

Fernandez, A.Z. Jr., DeMaria, E.J., Tichansky, D.S., et al. (2004) Experience with over 3,000 open and laparoscopic bariatric procedures: multivariate analysis of factors related to leak and resultant mortality. *Surgery and Endoscopy* 18: 193–197.

Fitzgerald, R., Saddler, M., Connolly, M., et al. (2014) Psoriasis and insulin resistance: a review. *Journal of Diabetes Research and Clinical Metabolism* http://www/hoajonline.com/journals/pdf2050-0866-3-3.pdf

Fiorentino, T.V., Prioletta, A., Zuo, P., et al. (2013) Hyperglycemia-induced oxidative stress and its role in diabetes mellitus related cardiovascular diseases. *Current Pharmaceutical Design* 19: 5695–5703.

Fisher, L., Mullan, J.T., Arean, P., et al. (2010) Diabetes distress but not clinical depression or depressive symptoms is associated with glycemic control in both cross-sectional and longitudinal analyses. *Diabetes Care* 33: 23–28.

Fortune, D.G., Richards, H.L., Kirby, B., et al. (2003) Psychological distress impairs clearance of psoriasis in patients treated with photochemotherapy. *Archive of Dermatology* 139:752–756.

Fortune, D.G., Richards, H.L., Main, C.J., et al. (2000) Pathological worrying, illness perceptions and disease severity in patients with psoriasis. *British Journal of Health Psychology* 5: 71–82.

Fortune, D.G., Richards, H.L., Main, C.J., et al. (1998) What patients with psoriasis believe about their condition. *Journal of the American Academy of Dermatology* 39: 196–201.

Freedland, K.E. (2004) Section II: Hypothesis 1: Depression is a risk factor for the development of Type 2 diabetes. *Diabetes Spectrum* 17: 150–152.

Frigg, A., Peterli, R., Peters, T., et al. (2004) Reduction in co-morbidities 4 years after laparoscopic adjustable gastric banding. *Obesity Surgery* 14(2): 216–223.

Furler, J., Kokanovic, R. (2010) Mental health: cultural competence. *Australian Family Physician* 39(4):206–208.

Furnes, B., Karin, G., Dysvik, E. (2014) Therapeutic elements in a self-management approach: experience from group participation among people suffering from chronic pain. *Patient Preference and Adherence* 8: 1089–1092.

Gale, L., Vedhara, K., Searle, A., et al. (2008) Patients' perspectives on foot complication in Type 2 diabetes: A qualitative study. *British Journal of General Practice.* doi: 10:3399/bjgp08X31957.

Garcia-Batista, Z.E., Guerra-Pena, K., Cano-Vindel, A. (2019) Validity and reliability of the Beck Depression Inventory (BDI-II) in the general and hospital population of the Dominican Republic. *PLos One* https://www.ncbi.nlm.nih.gov/pmc/articles/PMC6025862/

Gary, T.L., Crum, R.M., Cooper-Patrick, L., et al. (2000) Depressive symptoms and metabolic control in African-Americans with Type 2 diabetes. *Diabetes Care* 23(1): 23–29.

Gervey, B., Igou, E., Trope, Y. (2005) Positive mood and future-oriented self-evaluation. *Motivation and Emotion* 29: 267–294.

Giacco, F., Brownlee, M. (2010) Oxidative stress and diabetic complications. *Circulation Research* 107: 1058–1070.

Gill, D., Hatcher, S. (2000) Antidepressants for depression in medical illness [update software]. *Cochrane Database Systematic Review* (4): CD 001312.

Gobel-Fabbri, A.E., Fifkan, J., Franco, D., et al. (2008) Insulin restriction and associated morbidity and mortality in women with Type 1 diabetes. *Diabetes Care* 31(3): 415–419.

Gochman, D.S. (editor) (1997) *Handbook of Health Behavior Research.* New York: Plenum Press.

Goff, L.M., Moors, A., Harding, S, et al., (2020) Providing culturally sensitive diabetes self-management education and support for black African and Caribbean communities: a qualitative exploration of the challenges experienced by healthcare practitioners in inner London. *BMJ Open Diabetes Research and Care* 8(2) https://drc.bmj.com/content/8/2/e001818

Gold, A.E., Macleod, K.M., Frier, B.M. (1994) Frequency of severe hypoglycemia in patients with Type 1 diabetes with impaired awareness of hypoglycemia. *Diabetes Care* 17(7): 697–703.

Golden, S.H. (2012) Health disparities in endocrine disorders: biological, clinical, and non-clinical factors – an Endocrine Society scientific statement. *Journal of Clinical Endocrinology and Metabolism* 97(9): E1579–E1639.

Goldney, R.D., Phillips, P.J., Fisher, L.J. (2004) Diabetes, depression, and quality of life: a population study. *Diabetes Care* 27: 1066–1070.

Goodman, E., Whitaker, R.C. (2002) A prospective study of the role of depression in the development and persistence of adolescent obesity. *Pediatrics* 110(3): 497–504.

Gordon, K.B., Langley, R.G., Lenardi, C., et al. (2006) Clinical response to Adalimumab treatment in patients with moderate to severe psoriasis: double-blind, randomized controlled trial and open-label extension study. *Journal of the American Academy of Dermatology* 55: 598–606.

Gov UK. English Language Skills (2018. https://www.ethnicity-facts-figures. service.gov.uk/british-population/demographics/englishlanguage-skills/latest

Greco, D., Pisciotta, M., Gambina, F., et al. (2013) Celiac disease in subjects with Type 1 diabetes mellitus: a prevalence study in western Sicily (Italy). *Endocrine* 43(1): 108–111.

Grzywacz, J.G., Arcury, T.A., Edward, H., et al. (2011) Older adults common sense models of diabetes. *American Journal of Health Behaviour* 35(3): 318–333.

Guisado, J.A., Vaz, J.F., Alarcon, J., et al. (2002) Psychopathological status and interpersonal functioning following weight loss in morbidly obese patients undergoing bariatric surgery. *Obesity Surgery* 12(6): 835–840.

Gupta, M.A., Schork, N.J., Gupta, A.K., et al. (1993) Suicidal ideation in psoriasis. *International Journal of Dermatology* 32: 188–190.

Gutierrez, J., Long., J.A. (2011) Reliability and validity of diabetes specific health belief model scales in patients with diabetes and severe mental illness. *Diabetes Research and Clinical Practice* 92(3): 342–347.

Hadithi, M., de Boer, H., Meijer, J.W.R., et al. (2007) Coeliac disease in Dutch patients with Hashimoto's thyroiditis and vice-versa. *World Journal of Gastroenterology* 13(11): 1715–1722.

Hage, M., Zantout, M.S., Azar, S.I. (2011) Thyroid disorders and diabetes mellitus. *Journal of Thyroid Research* doi: 10:4061/2011/439463.

Hagger, M.S. (2013) The multiple pathways by which self-control predicts behavior. *Frontiers of Psychology* 4: 849.

Hajós, T.R., Polonsky, W.H., Pouwer, F., et al. (2014) Toward defining a cut-off score for elevated fear of hypoglycemia on the Hypoglycemia Fear Survey Worry subscale in patients with Type 2 diabetes. *Diabetes Care* 37(1):102–108.

Ham, J.A., Buck, K.D., Gonzalvo, J.D., et al. (2017) Clinical application of patient-centred diabetes care for people with serious mental illness. *Clinical Diabetes* 35(5): 313–320.

Hammes, H.P. (2003) Pathophysiological mechanisms of diabetic angiopathy. *Journal of Diabetes Complications* 17: 16–19.

Harder, H., Dinesen, B., Astrup, A. (2004) The effect of rapid weight loss on lipid profile and glycaemic control in obese Type 2 diabetic patients. *International Journal of Obesity* 28: 180–182.

Harris, R.H., Sasson, G., Mehler, P.S. (2013) Elevation of liver function tests in severe anorexia nervosa. *International Journal of Eating Disorders* 46: 369–374.

Hassmen, P., Koivula, N., Uutela, A. (2000) Physical exercise and psychological well-being: a population study in Finland. *Preventative Medicine* 30(1): 17–25.

Haviland, M.G., Dial, T.H., McGhee, W.H., et al. (2001) Depression and satisfaction with health plans. *Psychiatric Services* 52(3): 279.

Hemlock, C., Rosenthal, J.S., Winston, A. (1992) Fluoxetine-induced psoriasis. *Annals of Pharmacotherapy* 26: 211–212.

Hempler, N.F., Joensen, L.E., Willaing, I. (2016) Relationship between social network, social support and health behaviour in people with Type 1 and Type 2 diabetes: cross-sectional studies. *BMC Public Health* https://bmcpublichealth.biomedcentral.com/articles/10.1186/s12889-016-2819-1

Herrin, M. (2003) *Nutrition Counseling in the Treatment of Eating Disorders*. New York: Brunner-Routledge 3: 27–39.

Higgs, M.L., Wade, T., Cescato, M., et al. (1997) Differences between treatment seekers in an obese population: medical intervention vs. dietary restriction. *Journal of Behavioral Medicine* 20(4): 391–406.

Himmerich, H., Fulda, S., Linseisen, J., et al. (2008) Depression, comorbidities and the TNF-alpha system. *European Psychiatry* 23: 421–429.

Hirakawa, Y., Arima, H., Zoungas, S., et al. (2014) Impact of visit-to-visit glycemic variability on the risks of macrovascular and microvascular events and all-cause mortality in Type 2 diabetes: the ADVANCE trial. *Diabetes Care* 37: 2359–2365.

Hoban, C., Sareen, J., Henriksen, C.A., et al. (2015) Mental health associated with foot complications of diabetes mellitus. *Elsevier* https://www.sciencedirect.com/science/article/abs/pii/S1268773114001180

Höke, U., Thijssen, J., Bommel, R van V., et al. (2013) Influence of diabetes on left ventricular systolic and diastolic function and on long-term outcome after cardiac resynchronization therapy. *Diabetes Care* 36(4): 985–991.

Holford, P. (2011) *Say No to Diabetes: 10 Secrets to Preventing and Reversing Diabetes*. London: Piatkus, Little, Brown Book Group.

Holmes, S.R., Gudridge, T.A., Gaudiani, J.L. (2012) Dysphagia in severe anorexia nervosa and potential therapeutic intervention: a case series. *Annuls of Otology, Rhinology and Laryngology* 121: 449–456.

Holt, R.I., de Groot, M., Lucki, I., et al. (2014) NIDDK international conference report on diabetes and depression: current understanding and future directions. *Diabetes Care* 37: 2067–2077.

Horne, R. (1997) Representation of medicine and treatment: advances in theory and measurement. In: Petrie, K.J., Weinmann, J. (Eds.) *Perceptions of Health and Illness: Current Research and Applications*. London: Harwood Academic, 155–188.

Horner, R.L. (2012) Neural control of the upper airway: integrative physiological mechanisms and relevance for sleep disordered breathing. *Comprehensive Physiology* 2: 479–535.

Hood, K.K., Hilliard, M., Piatt, G., et al. (2018) Effective strategies for encouraging behaviour change in people with diabetes. *Diabetes Management (London)* 5(6): 499–510.

Hsia, Y-T., Cheng, W-C., Liao, W-C., et al. (2015) Type 1 diabetes and increased risk of subsequent asthma: a nationwide population-based cohort study. *Medicine* 94(36): pe1466.

Hsu, Y.Y., Chen, B.H., Huang, M.C., et al. (2009) Disturbed eating behaviour in Taiwanese adolescents with Type 1 diabetes mellitus: A comparative study. *Pediatric Diabetes* 10: 74–81.

Hu, T., Zhang, D., Wang, J., et al. (2014) Relation between emotion regulation and mental health: a meta-analysis review. *Psychological Report* 114: 341–362.

Huston, S.A., Houk, C.P. (2011) Common Sense model of illness in youth with Type 1 diabetes or Sickle Cell disease. *Journal of Paediatric Pharmacology and Therapy* 16(4): 270–280.

Iglay, K., Hannachi, H., Joseph, H.P., et al. (2016) Prevalence and co-prevalence of comorbidities among patients with Type 2 diabetes mellitus. *Current Medical Research and Opinion* 32(7): 1243–1252. doi:10.1185/03007995.2016.1168291

Ikeda, R.M., Kresnow, M.J., Mercy, J.A., et al. (2001) Medical conditions and nearly lethal suicide attempts. *Suicide and Life-Threatening Behaviour* 32: 60–67.

Illman, J., Corringham, R., Robinson, D. Jr., et al. (2005) Are inflammatory cytokines the common link between cancer-associated cachexia and depression? *Journal of Support Oncology* 3: 37–50.

Inagaki, T., Yamamoto, M., Tsubouchi, K., et al. (2003) Echocardiographic investigation of pericardial effusion in a case of anorexia nervosa. *International Journal of Eating Disorders* 33: 364–366.

International Diabetes Federation – IDF (2015) Brussels, Belgium: International Diabetes Federation. http://www.diabetesatlas.org

Ismail, K., Winkley, K., Stahl, D., et al. (2007) A cohort study of people with diabetes and their first foot ulcer: the role of depression on mortality. *Diabetes Care* 30(6): 1473–1479.

Izard, C.E. (2007) Basic emotions, natural kinds, emotion schemas, and a new paradigm. *Perspectives on Psychological Science* 2: 260–280.

Jackson, J.L., Kroenke, K. (1999) Difficult patient encounters in the ambulatory clinic: clinical predictors and outcomes. *Archive of Internal Medicine* 159(10): 1069–1075.

Jaremka, L.M., Lindgren, M.E., Kiecolt-Glaser, J.K. (2013) Synergistic relationships among stress, depression, and troubled relationships: insights from psychoneuroimmunology. *Depression and Anxiety* 30: 288–296.

Jarvholm, K., Olbers, T., Marcus, C., et al. (2012) Short-term psychological outcomes in severely obese adolescents after bariatric surgery. *Obesity* 20(2): 318–323.

Jaser, S.S., Patel, N., Rothman, R.L., et al. (2014) A randomized pilot of a positive psychology intervention to improve adherence in adolescents with Type 1 diabetes. *Diabetes Educator* 40: 659–667.

Jehle, P.M., Jehle, D.R., Mohan, S., et al. (1998) Serum levels of insulin-like growth factor system components and relationship to bone metabolism in Type I and Type 2 diabetes mellitus patients. *Journal of Endocrinology* 159: 297–306.

Jensen, P., Thyssen, J.P., Zachariae, C., et al. (2013) Cardiovascular risk factors in subjects with psoriasis: a cross-sectional general population study. *International Journal of Dermatology* 52: 681–583.

Johnston, A., Arnadottir, S., Gudjonsson, J.E., et al. (2008) Obesity in psoriasis: leptin and resistin as mediators of cutaneous inflammation. *British Journal of Dermatology* 159: 342–350.

Jonas, B.S., Mussolino, M.E. (2000) Symptoms of depression as a prospective risk factor for stroke. *Psychosomatic Medicine* 62(4): 463–471.

Kalarchian, M.A., Marcus, M.D., Levine, M.D., et al. (2007) Psychiatric disorders among bariatric surgery candidates: relationship to obesity and functional health status. *American Journal of Psychiatry* 164(2): 328–334.

Kamal, N., Chami, T., Andersen, A. (1991) Delayed gastrointestinal transit times in anorexia nervosa and bulimia nervosa. *Gastroenterology* 101:1320–1324.

Karadag, A.S., Yavuz, B., Ertugrul, D.T., et al. (2010) Is psoriasis a pre-atherosclerotic disease? Increased insulin resistance and impaired endothelial function in patients with psoriasis. *International Journal of Dermatology* 49: 642–646.

Karim, M., Araban, M., Zareban, I., et al. (2016) Determinants of adherence to self-care behaviour among young women with Type 2 diabetes: an explanation based on health belief model. *Medical Journal of the Islamic Republic of Iran* 30: 368.

Karter, A.J., Stevens, M.R., Brown, A.F., et al. (2007) Educational disparities in health behaviors among patients with diabetes: The Translating Research Into Action for Diabetes (TRIAD) Study. *BMC Public Health* 7: 308.

Kastner, S., Salbach-Andrae, H., Renneberg, B. (2012) Echocardiographic findings in adolescents with anorexia nervosa at beginning of treatment and after weight recovery. *European Child and Adolescent Psychiatry* 21: 15–21.

Katon, W.J. (2003) Clinical and health service relationships between major depression, depressive symptoms, and general medical illness. *Biological Psychiatry* 54: 216–226.

Katsilambros, N., Kanka-Gantenbein, C., Liatis, S., et al. (2011) *Diabetic Emergencies and Clinical Management.* Chichester, West Sussex: Wiley-Blackwell.

Keating, S.T., Plutsky, J., El-Osta, A. (2016) Epigenetic changes in diabetes and cardiovascular risk. *Circulation Research* 118: 1706–1722.

Keidar, A. (2011) Bariatric surgery for Type 2 diabetes reversal: the risks. *Diabetes Care* 34(2): S361–S367.

Keidar, A., Appelbaum, L., Schweiger, C., et al. (2010) Dilated upper sleeve gastrectomy can be associated with severe postoperative gastroesophageal dysmotility and reflux. *Obesity Surgery* 20: 140–147.

Keidar, A., Szold, A., Carmon, E., et al. (2005) Band slippage after laparoscopic adjustable gastric banding: etiology and treatment. *Surgical Endoscopy* 19: 262–267.

Kelly, S.D., Howe, C.J., Hendler, J.P., et al. (2005) Disordered eating behaviors in youth with Type 1 diabetes. *Diabetes Educator* 34: 572–583.

Kessing, L.V., Nilsson, F.M., Siersma, V., et al. (2004) Increased risk of developing diabetes in depressive and bipolar disorders? *Journal of Psychiatric Research* 38: 395–402.

Kimball, A.B., Yu, A.P., Signorovitch. J., et al. (2012) The effects of adalimumab treatment and psoriasis severity on self-reported work productivity and activity impairment for patients with moderate to severe psoriasis. *Journal of the American Academy of Dermatology* 66: e67–e76.

176   *References*

Kinzl, J.F., Traweger, C., Trefalt, E., et al. (2013) Psychosocial consequences of weight loss following gastric banding for morbid obesity. *Obesity Surgery* 13(1): 105–110.

Kirk, J.K., Graves, D.E., Bell, R.A., et al. (2007) Racial and ethnic disparities in self-monitoring of blood glucose among US adults: a qualitative review. *Ethnic Disorders* 17(1): 135–142.

Klein, J.P., Waxman, S.G. (2003) The brain in diabetes: molecular changes in neurons and their implications for end-organ damage. *Lancet Neurology* 2: 548–554.

Kim, R.P., Edelman, S.V., Kim, D.D. (2001) Musculoskeletal complications of diabetes mellitus. *Clinical Diabetes* 19(3): 132–135.

Kjeldsen, S.E., Hedner, T., Jamerson, K., et al. (1998) Hypertension Optimal Treatment (HOT) Study. *Hypertension* 31(4): 1014–1020.

Klok, M.D., Jakobsdottir, S., Drent, M.L. (2007) The role of leptin and ghrelin in the regulation of food intake and body weight in humans: a review. *Obesity Review* 8: 21–34.

Koubaa, S., Hallstrom, T., Lindholm, C. (2005) Pregnancy and neonatal outcomes in women with eating disorders. *Obstetrics* & Gynaecology 105: 255–260.

Kubik, J.F., Gill, R.S., Laffin, M., et al. (2013) The impact of bariatric surgery on psychological health. *Journal of Obesity*. 10.1155/2013/837989

Kuna, S.T., Reboussin, D.M., Borradaile, K.E., et al. (2013) Long-term effect of weight loss on obstructive sleep apnoea severity in obese patients with Type 2 diabetes. *Sleep* 36:641–649.

Kurd, S.K., Troxel, A.B., Crits-Christoph, P., et al. (2010) The risk of depression, anxiety, and suicidality in patients with psoriasis: a population-based cohort study. *Archive of Dermatology* 146: 891–895.

Koronouri, O., Maguire, A.M., Knip, M., et al. (2009) Other complications and conditions associated with diabetes in children and adolescents. *Journal of Pediatric Diabetes*. 10(12): 204–210.

Kraeft, J.J., Uppot, R.N., Heffess, A.M. (2013) Imaging findings in eating disorders. *American Journal of Research/American Journal of Roentgenology* 200: W328–W335.

Kung, H.C., Hoyert, D.L., Xu, J.Q., et al. (2008) Deaths: final data for 2005. *National Vital Statistics Reports* 56(10) http://www.cdc.gov/nchs/data/nvsr/nvsr56/nvsr56_10.pdf

Kurian, A.K., Cardarelli, K.M. (2007) Racial and ethnic differences in cardiovascular disease risk factors: a systematic review. *Ethnic Disorders* 17(1): 143–152.

Laake, J.P., Stahl, D., Amiel, S.A., et al. (2014) The association between depressive symptoms and systemic inflammation in people with Type 2 diabetes: findings from the South London Diabetes Study. *Diabetes Care* 37: 2186–2192.

Lai, Y., Wang, J., Jiang, F., et al. (2011) The relationship between serum thyrotropin and components of metabolic syndrome. *Endocrine Journal* 58(1): 23–30.

Larger, E. (2005) Weight gain & insulin treatment. *Diabetes Metabolism* 31: 4S51–4S56.

Lauret, E., Rodrigo, L. (2013) Celiac disease and autoimmune-associated conditions. *Biomedical Research International*. 10.1155/2013/127589.

Lavda, A.C., Webb, T.L., Thompson, A.R. (2012) A meta-analysis of the effectiveness of psychological interventions for adults with skin conditions. *British Journal of Dermatology* 167: 970–979.

Law, G.U., Kelly, T.P., Huey, D., et al. (2002). Self-management and well-being in adolescents with diabetes mellitus: Do illness representations play a regulatory role? *Journal of Adolescent Health* 31(4): 381–385.

Lazaro, L., Andres, S., Calvo, A., et al. (2013) Normal gray and white matter volume after weight restoration in adolescents with anorexia nervosa. *International Journal of Eating Disorders* 46: 481–488.

Leeds, J.S., Hopper, A.D., Hadjivassiliou, M., et al. (2011) High prevalence of microvascular complications in adults with Type 1 diabetes and newly diagnosed celiac disease. *Diabetes Care* 34(10): 2158–2163.

Lehmer, L.M., Ragsdale, B.D. (2012) Calcified periarthritis: more than a shoulder problem. *The Journal of Bone and Joint Surgery in America* 94(21): e157.

Lehrer, P.M., Feldman, J., Giardino, N., et al. (2002) Psychological aspects of asthma. *Journal of Consulting Clinical Psychology* 70: 691–711.

Leventhal, H., Nerenz, D. R., Steele, D. J. (1984) Illness representations and coping with health threats. In A. Baum, S. E. Taylor & J. E. Singer (Eds.), *Handbook of Psychology and Health* (Vol. IV Social psychological aspects of health, pp. 219–252). Hillsdale, NJ: Lawrence Erlbaum.

Leventhal, H., Meyer, D., Nerenz, D. (1980) The common sense representation of illness danger. In: S. Rachman (Ed.), *Contributions to Medical Psychology* (Vol. 2, pp. 7–30). Oxford, UK: Pergamon Press.

Leventhal, H. (1970) Findings and theory in the study of fear communications. *Advances in Experimental Social Psychology* 5: 119–186.

Li, C., Ford, E.S., Guixiang, Z, et al. (2010) Undertreatment of mental health problems in adults with diagnosed diabetes and serious psychological distress: the behavioral risk factor surveillance system, 2007. *Diabetes Care* 33(5): 1061–1064.

Litwak, L., Goh, S-Y., Hussein, Z., et al. (2013) Prevalence of diabetes complications in people with Type 2 diabetes mellitus and its association with baseline characteristics in the multinational Archive study. *Diabetology and Metabolic Syndrome* 5(57): http://www.dmsjournal.com/content/5/1/57

Lombardi, F., Franzese, A., Lafusco, D., et al. (2010) Bone involvement in clusters of autoimmune diseases: just a complication? *Bone* 46(2): 551–555.

Lo Sauro, C., Ravaldi, C., Cabras, P.L. (2008) Stress, hypothalamic-pituitary-adrenal axis and eating disorder. *Neuropsychobiology* 57: 95–115.

Löwe, B., Zipfel, S., Buchholz, C., et al. (2001) Long-term outcome of anorexia nervosa in a prospective 21-year follow-up study. *Psychology Medicine* 31: 881–890.

Ludvigsson, J.F., Ludvigsson, J., Ekbom, A., et al. (2006) Celiac disease and risk of subsequent Type 1 diabetes: a general population cohort study of children and adolescents. *Diabetes Care* 29(11): 2483–2488.

Lustman, P.J., Clouse, R.E., Nix, B.D., et al. (2006) Sertraline for prevention of depression recurrence in diabetes: a randomized, double-blind, placebo-controlled trial. *Archive of General Psychiatry* 63(5): 521–529.

Lustman, P.J., Clouse, R.E., Ciechanowski, P.S., et al. (2005) Depression-related hyperglycemia in Type 1 diabetes: a meditational approach. *Psychosomatic Medicine* 67: 195–199.

Lustman, P.J., Clouse, R.E. (2002) Treatment of depression in diabetes: impact on mood and medical outcome. *Journal of Psychosomatic Research* 53: 917–924.

Lustman, P.J., Anderson, R.J., Freedland, K.E., et al. (2000a) Depression and poor glycaemic control: a meta-analytic review of the literature. *Diabetes Care* 23: 434–442.

Lustman, P.J., Freedland, K.E., Griffith, L.S., et al. (2000b) Fluoxetine for depression in diabetes: a randomized double-blind placebo controlled trial. *Diabetes Care* 23(5): 618–623.

Lustman, P.J., Clouse, R.E., Griffith, L.S., et al. (1997a) Screening for depression in diabetes using the Beck Depression Inventory. *Psychosomatic Medicine* 59: 24–31.

Lustman, P.J., Griffith, L.S., Freedland, K.E., et al. (1997b) The course of major depression in diabetes. *General Hospital Psychiatry* 19(2): 138–143.

Lustman, P.J., Griffith, L.S., Clouse, R.E., et al. (1997c) Effects of Nortriptyline on depression and glycemic control in diabetes: results of a double-blind, placebo-controlled trial. *Psychosomatic Medicine* 59: 241–250.

Lyoo, I.K., Yoon, S., Jacobson, A.M., et al. (2012) Prefrontal cortical deficits in Type 1 diabetes mellitus: brain correlates of comorbid depression. *Archives of General Psychiatry* 69: 1267–1276.

MacRury, S., Stephen, K., Main, F., et al. (2018) Reducing amputations in people with diabetes (RAPID): Evaluation of a new care pathway. *International Journal of Environmental Research in Public Health* 15(5): 999.

Mafauzy, M., Mohammed, W.B., Anum, M.Y., et al. (1990) A study of the fasting diabetic patient during the month of Ramadan. *Medical Journal of Malaysia* 45: 14–17.

Malone, J.I., Hansen. B.C. (2019) Does obesity cause Type 2 diabetes mellitus (T2DM)? Or is it the opposite? *Pediatric Diabetes* 20(1): 5–9.

Mamplekou, E., Komesidou, V., Bissias, C., et al. (2005) Psychological condition and quality of life in patients with morbid obesity before and after surgical weight loss. *Obesity Surgery* 15(8): 1177–1184.

Mannucci, I., Rotella, F., Ricca, V., et al. (2005) Eating disorders in patients with Type 1 diabetes: a meta-analysis. *Journal of Endocrinological Investigation* 28: 417–419.

Maratou, E., Hadjidakis, D.J., Kollias, A., et al. (2009) Studies of insulin resistance in patients with clinical and subclinical hypothyroidism. *European Journal of Endocrinology* 160(5): 785–790.

Marianna, R., Olga, B., Tzvi, B., et al. (2006) TH1/TH2 cytokine balance in patients with both Type 1 diabetes mellitus and asthma. *Cytokine* 34:170–176.

Marinari, G.M., Papadia, F.S., Briatore, L. (2006) Type 2 diabetes and weight loss following biliopancreatic diversion for obesity. *Obesity Surgery* 16: 1440–1444.

Markowitz, J.T., Butler, D.A., Volkening, L.K., et al. (2010) Brief screening tool for disordered eating in diabetes: internal consistency and external validity in a contemporary sample of pediatric patients with type 1 diabetes. *Diabetes Care* 33: 495–500.

Marliss, E.B., Vranic, M. (2002) Insulin release and its role in glucoregulation: Implications for diabetes. *Diabetes* 51(1): S271–S283.

Maslow, A.H. (1943) A theory of human motivation. *Psychology Revisited* 50: 370.

Mayo Clinic (2018) Electro-convulsive therapy (ECT) https://www.mayoclinic.org/tests-procedures/electroconvulsive-therapy/about/pac-20393894

Mayer-Davis, E.J., Sparks, K.C., Hirst, K., et al. (2004) Dietary intake in the diabetes prevention program cohort: baseline and 1-year post-randomisation. *Annals of Epidemiology* 14: 763–772.

McAndrew, L. M., Crede, M., Maestro, K., et al. (2019). Using the common sense model to understand health outcomes for medically unexplained symptoms: A meta-analysis. *Health Psychology Review*. doi: 10.1080/17437199.2018.1521730

McCrimmon, R.J., Ryan, C.M., Frier, B.M. (2012) Diabetes and cognitive dysfunction. *Lancet.* 379(9833): 2291. https://journals.plos.org/plosone/article?id=10.1371/journal.pone.0157268

McKellar, J.D., Piette, J.D., Humphreys, K. (2004) Does self-care adherence mediate the relationship between depression and subsequent diabetes symptoms? *The Diabetes Educator* 30(3): 485–491.

Mc Sharry, J., Moss-Morris, R., Kendrick, T. (2011) Illness perceptions and glycaemic control in diabetes: a systematic review with meta-analysis. *Diabetic Medicine* 28: 1300–1310.

Mehler, P.S., Brown, C. (2015) Anorexia nervosa – medical complications. *Journal of Eating Disorders* http://www.jeatdisord.com/content/3/1/11

Mehler, P.S., Sabel, A.L., Watson, T., et al. (2008) High risk of osteoporosis in male patients with eating disorders. *International Journal of Eating Disorders* 41: 666–672.

Mehta, N.N., Azfar, R.S., Shin, D.B., et al. (2010) Patients with severe psoriasis are at increased risk of cardiovascular mortality: cohort study using the General Practice Research Database. *European Heart Journal* 31: 1000–1006.

Meloni, A., Mandas, C., Jores, R.D., et al. (2009) Prevalence of autoimmune thyroiditis in children with celiac disease and effect of gluten withdrawal. *The Journal of Pediatrics*, 155(1): 51–55.

Mertens, V.C., Bosma, H., Groffen, D.A., et al. (2012) Good friends, high income or resilience? What matters most for elderly patients? *European Journal of Public Health* 22: 666–671.

Meltzer, D., Egleston, B. (2000) How patients with diabetes perceive their risk for major complications. *Effective Clinical Practice* 3(1): 7–15.

Michie, S., Atkins, L., West, R. (2014) *The Behaviour Change Wheel. A Guide to Designing Interventions*. Silverback Publishing.

Miller, K.K., Grinspoon, S.K., Ciampa, J. (2005) Medical findings in outpatients with anorexia nervosa. *Archive of Intern Medicine*. 165: 561–566.

Mitchell, J.E., Crosby, R., de Zwaan, M., et al. (2013) Possible risk factors for increased suicide following bariatric surgery. *Obesity* https://www.ncbi.nlm.nih.gov/pmc/articles/PMC4372842/

Misra-Hebert, A.D., Isaacson, J.H. (2012) Overcoming health care disparities via better cross-cultural communication and health literacy. *Cleveland Clinic Journal of Medicine*. 79(2): 127–133.

180   References

Misra, M., Klibanski, A. (2014) Anorexia nervosa and bone. *Journal of Endocrinology* 221: R163–R176.

Misra, D.P., Das, S., Sahu, P.K. (2012) Prevalence of inflammatory markers (high-sensitivity C-reactive protein, nuclear factorκB, and adiponectin) in Indian patients with Type 2 diabetes mellitus with and without macrovascular complications. *Metabolic Syndrome Related Disorder* 10: 209–213.

Moffitt, T.E., Arseneault, L., Belsky, D., et al. (2011) A gradient of childhood self-control predicts health, wealth, and public safety. *Proceedings of the National Academy of Science* 108: 2693-2698.

Monnier, L., Mas, E., Ginet, C., et al. (2006) Activation of oxidative stress by acute glucose fluctuations compared with sustained chronic hyperglycemia in patients with Type 2 diabetes. *Journal of the American Medical Association* 295: 1681–1687.

Morris, L.G., Stephenson, K.E., Herring, S. (2004) Recurrent acute pancreatitis in anorexia and bulimia. *Journal of Physiology* 5: 231–234.

Morrisson, E.L. (2012) Diabetes and eating disorders: together they're linked with a double dose of health consequences. *Today's Dietician* 14(12): 40–44.

Moss-Morris, R., Weinman, J., Petrie, K. J., et al. (2002) The revised Illness Perception Questionnaire (IPQ-R). *Psychology and Health* 17(1): 1–16.

Muntner, P., Carey, R.M., Gidding, S., et al. (2018) Potential US Population Impact of the 2017 ACC/AHA High Blood Pressure Guideline. *Circulation* 137: 109.

Muraven, M., Gagné, M., Rosman, H. (2008) Helpful self-control: Autonomy support, vitality, and depletion. *Journal of Experimental Social Psychology* 44: 573–585.

Musselman, D.L., Betan, E., Larsen, H., et al. (2003) Relationship of depression to diabetes Types 1 and 2: epidemiology, biology, and treatment. *Biological Psychiatry* 54: 317–329.

Myhre, A.G., Aarsetøy, H., Undlien, D.E., et al. (2013) High frequency of coeliac disease among patients with autoimmune adrenocortical failure. *Scandinavian Journal of Gastroenterology* 38(5): 511–515.

Myers, D.G. (2000) The funds, friends, and faith of happy people. *American Psychology* 55: 56–67.

Nalysnyk, L., Hernandez-Medina, M., Krishnarajah, G. (2010) Glycaemic variability and complications in patients with diabetes mellitus: evidence from a systematic review of the literature. *Diabetes, Obesity and Metabolism* 12: 288–298.

National Eating Disorders Association (2021) Statistics and research on eating disorders https://www.nationaleatingdisorders.org/statistics-research-eating-disorders

National Collaboration Centre for Primary Care (2008) Medicines concordance and adherence involving adults and carers in decisions about prescribed medicines. National Collaboration Centre for Primary Care.

National Health Service (2000) *NHS Plan 2000*. London: Department of Health.

National Health Service (2018) Overview: Addison's disease. https://www.nhs.uk/conditions/addisonsdisease/#:~:text=About%208%2C400%20people%20in%20the, common%20in%20women%20than%20men

References   181

National Institute for Health (2017) Diabetes in children and teens: symptoms and diagnosis. https://www.medicalnewstoday.com/articles/284974#:~:text=How%20does %20diabetes%20aff ect%20children%20and%20teens%3F&text=In%202017%2C%20the %20National%20Institutes,type%202%20by%204.8%20percent

National Institute for Health and Care Excellence (NICE) (2014a) *The management of Type 2 diabetes.* London: NICE. nice.org.uk/cg87

National Institute for Health and Care Excellence (NICE) (2014b) Press release: NICE updates weight-loss surgery criteria for people with Type 2 diabetes. nice. org.uk/cg190

National Institute for Health and Care Excellence (NICE) (2014c) *Obesity Identification Assessment and Management of Overweight and Obesity in Children, Young People and Adults.* nice.org.uk/cg189

National Institute for Health and Clinical Excellence (NICE) (2004) *Eating Disorders. Core Interventions in the Treatment of and Management of Anorexia Nervosa, Bulimia Nervosa and Related Eating Disorders.* National Institute for Clinical Excellence, Clinical Guideline 9. http://guidance.nice.org.uk

Naylor, C., Galea, A., Parsonage, M., et al. (2012) Long-term conditions and mental health: the cost of co-morbidities. *The King's Fund.*

Niego, S.H., Kofman, M.D., Weiss, J.J., et al. (2007) Binge eating in the bariatric surgery population: a review of the literature. *International Journal of Eating Disorders* 40(4): 349–359.

Neimann, A.L., Shin, D.B., Wang, X., et al. (2006) Prevalence of cardiovascular risk factors in patients with psoriasis. *Journal of American Academic Dermatology* 55: 829–835.

Neilsen, S., Emborg, C., Molbak, A-G. (2002) Mortality in concurrent Type 1 diabetes and anorexia nervosa. *Diabetes Care* 25(2): 309–312.

Netzel, P.J., Mueller, P.S., Rummans, T.A., et al. (2002) Safety, efficacy, and effects on glycemic control of electroconvulsive therapy in insulin-requiring Type 2 diabetic patients. *Journal of Electroconvulsive Therapy* 18: 16–21.

Neuhausen, S.L., Steele, S., Ryan, S., et al. (2008) Co-occurrence of celiac disease and other autoimmune diseases in celiacs and their first-degree relatives. *Journal of Autoimmunity* 31 (2): 160–165.

Neumark-Sztainer, D., Patterson, J., Mellin, A., et al. (2002) Weight control practices and disordered eating behaviours among adolescent females and males with Type 1 diabetes: associations with socio-demographics, weight concerns, familial factors and metabolic outcomes. *Diabetes Care* 25: 1289–1296.

Nuevo, R., Chatterji, S., Fraguas, D., et al. (2011) Increased risk of diabetes mellitus among persons with psychotic symptoms: Results from the WHO World Health Survey. *Journal of Clinical Psychiatry* 72: 1592–1599.

Nicolucci, A., Burns, K., Holt, R.I., et al. (2013) Diabetes Attitudes, Wishes and Needs second study (DAWN2): cross-national benchmarking of diabetes-related psychosocial outcomes for people with diabetes. *Diabetes Medicine* 30: 767–777.

O'Brien, J.P.E., Dixon, J.B., Laurie, C., et al. (2006) Treatment of mild to moderate obesity with laparoscopic adjustable gastric banding or an intensive medical program: a randomized trial. *Annals of Internal Medicine* 144(9): 625–633.

O'Leary, C., Walsh, C.H., Wieneke, P., et al. (2002) Coeliac disease and auto-immune Addison's disease: a clinical pitfall. *Monthly Journal of the Association of Physicians* 95(2): 79–82.

Obesity Health Alliance (2017) The cost of obesity. http://obesityhealthalliance.org.uk/wp-content/uploads/2017/10/OHA-briefing-paper-Costs-of-Obesity-.pdf

Oftedal, B.F. (2011) *Motivation for self-management among adults with Type 2 diabetes.* University of Stavanger, Norway.

Ogden, J. (2016) Celebrating variability and a call to limit systematisation: the example of the Behaviour Change Technique Taxonomy and the Behaviour Change Wheel. *Health Psychology Review* 10: 245–250.

Orbell, S., Phillips, L. A. (2019). Automatic processes and self-regulation of illness. *Health Psychology Review.* doi: 10.1080/17437199.2018.1503559.

Paddison, C.A.M. (2010). Exploring physical and psychological wellbeing among adults with Type 2 diabetes: Identifying a need to improve the experiences of Pacific peoples. *New Zealand Medical Journal* 123(1310).

Park, M., Katon, W.J., Wolf, F.M. (2013) Depression and risk of mortality in individuals with diabetes: a meta-analysis and systematic review. *General Hospital Psychiatry* 35: 217–225.

Paschalides, C., Wearden, A. J., Dunkerley, R., et al. (2004). The associations of anxiety, depression and personal illness representations with glycaemic control and health-related quality of life in patients with Type 2 diabetes mellitus. *Journal of Psychosomatic Research* 57(6), 557–564.

Patel, N.R., Chew-Graham, C., Bundy, C., et al. (2015) Illness beliefs and the sociocultural context of diabetes self-management in British south Asians: a mixed-method study. *BMC Family Practice* https://bmcfampract.biomedcentral.com/articles/10.1186/s12875-015-0269-y

Pavy, F.W. (1885) Introductory address to the discussion of the clinical aspects of glycosuria. *Lancet* 2: 1085–1087.

Peveler, R.C., Carson, A., Rodin, G. (2002) Depression in medical patients. *British Medical Journal* 325: 149–152.

Penckofer, S., Quinn, L., Byrn, M., et al. (2012) Does glycemic variability impact mood and quality of life? *Diabetes and Technological Therapy* 14: 303–310.

Penno, G., Solini, A., Bonora, E., et al. (2013) HbA1c variability as an independent correlate of nephropathy, but not retinopathy, in patients with Type 2 diabetes: The Renal Insufficiency And Cardiovascular Events (RIACE) Italian multicenter study. *Diabetes Care* 36: 2301–2310.

Peterhansel, C., Petroff, D., Klinitzke, G., et al. (2013) Risk of completed suicide after bariatric surgery: a systematic review. *Obesity Reviews* https://www.ncbi.nlm.nih.gov/books/NBK142927/

Petty, R., Sensky, T., Mahler, R. (1991) Diabetologists' assessments of their out-patients' emotional state and health beliefs: accuracy and possible sources of bias. *Psychotherapy and Psychosomatics* 55(2–4): 164–169.

Perrin, N.E., Davis, M.J., Robertson, N., et al. (2017) The prevalence of diabetes-specific emotional distress in people with Type 2 diabetes: a systematic review and meta-analysis. *Diabetes Medicine* 34(11): 1508–1520.

Peters G.-J.Y., Kok, G. (2016) All models are wrong, but some are useful: a comment on Ogden, 2016). *Health Psychology Review* 10: 265–268.

Peveler, R.C., Bryden, K.S., Neil, A.W., et al. (2005) The relationship of disordered eating habits and attitudes to clinical outcomes in young adult females with Type 1 diabetes. *Diabetes Care* 28(1): 84–88.

Poraira, R.F., Alvarenga, M. (2007) Disordered eating: identifying, treating, preventing, and differentiating it from eating disorders. *Diabetes Spectrum* 20(3): 140–146.

Peyrot, M., Kovacs-Burns, K., Davies, M., et al. (2013) Diabetes Attitudes, Wishes and Needs 2 (DAWN2): A multinational, multi-stakeholder study of psychosocial and person-centred diabetes care. *Science Direct* https://www.sciencedirect.com/science/article/pii/S0168822712004809

Peyrot, M., Rubin, R. R., Lauritzen, T., et al. (2005). Psychosocial problems and barriers to improved diabetes management: Results of the cross-national Diabetes Attitudes, Wishes and Needs (DAWN) Study. *Diabetic Medicine* 22(10): 1379–1385.

Peyrot, M., Rubin, R.R. (1997) Levels and risks of depression and anxiety symptomology among diabetic adults. *Diabetes Care* 20: 585–590.

Pham-Short, A., Donaghue, K.C., Ambler, G., et al. (2010) Coeliac disease in Type 1 diabetes from 1990 to 2009: higher incidence in young children after longer diabetes duration. *Diabetic Medicine* 29(9): e.286–e.289.

Picot, J., Jones, J., Colquitt, J.L., et al. (2009) The clinical effectiveness and cost-effectiveness of bariatric (weight loss) surgery for obesity: a systematic review and economic evaluation. *Health Technology Assessment* 13(41): 1–190, 215–357.

Piette, J.D., Richardson, C., Valenstein, M. (2004) Addressing the needs of patients with multiple chronic illness: the case of diabetes and depression. *The American Journal of Managed Care* 10(2): 152–164.

Piette, J.D., Schillinger, D., Potter, M.B., et al. (2003) Dimensions of patient-provider communication and diabetes self-care in an ethnically-diverse population. *Journal of General Internal Medicine* 18: 1–10.

Pinhas-Hamlet, O., Levy-Shraga, Y. (2013) Eating disorders in adolescents with Type 1 and Type 2 diabetes. *Current Diabetes Reports* 12: 289–297.

Podnos, Y.D., Jimenez, J.C., Wilson, S.E., et al. (2003) Complications after laparoscopic gastric bypass: a review of 3,464 cases. *Archives of Surgery* 138: 957–961.

Ponder, S.W. (2017) Hyperthyroidism and Type 1 diabetes. https://www.sugarsurfing.com/single-post/2017/02/09/Hyperthyroidism-and-type-1-diabetes

Pop-Bisui, R. (2010) Cardiac autonomic neuropathy in diabetes. *Diabetes Care* 33(2): 434–441.

Porcelli, P., Leandro, G., De Carne, M. (1998) Functional gastrointestinal disorders and eating disorders. Relevance of the association in clinical management. *Scandinavian Journal of Gastroenterology* 33: 577–582.

Pound, N., Chipchase, S., Treece, K., et al. (2005) Ulcer-free survival following management of foot ulcers in diabetes. *Diabetes Medicine* 22(10): 1306–1309.

Pouwer, F., Beekman, A.T., Lubach, C., et al. (2006) Nurses' recognition and registration of depression, anxiety and diabetes-specific emotional problems in outpatients with diabetes mellitus. *Patient Education and Counseling* 60(2): 235–240.

Pouwer, F., Beekman, A.T., Nijpels, G., et al. (2003) Rates and risks for co-morbid depression in patients with Type 2 diabetes mellitus: results from a community-based study. *Diabetologia*. 46(7): 892–898.

Prochaska, J.O., Velicer, W.F. (1997) The Transtheoretical Model of health behaviour change. *American Journal of Health Promotion* 12: 38–48.

Ramasubbu, R. (2002) Insulin resistance: a metabolic link between depressive disorder and atherosclerotic vascular diseases. *Medical Hypotheses* 59: 537–551.

Reiter, J., Wexler, I.D., Shehadeh, N., et al. (2007) Type 1 diabetes and prolonged fasting. *Diabetic Medicine* 24: 436–439.

Rendell, M. (2004) The role of sulphonylureas in the management of Type 2 diabetes mellitus. *Drugs* 64: 1339–1358.

Retnakaran, R., Zinman, B. (2009) Thiazolidinediones and clinical outcomes in Type 2 diabetes. *Lancet* 373: 2088–2090.

Revicki, D.A., Menter, A., Feldman, S., et al. (2008) Adalimumab improves health-related quality of life in patients with moderate to severe plaque psoriasis compared with the United States general population norms: results from a randomized, controlled Phase III study. *Health Quality and Life Outcomes* 6: 75.

Robertson, S.M., Amspoker, A.B., Cully, J.A., et al. (2013) Affective symptoms and change in diabetes self-efficacy and glycaemic control. *Diabetes Medicine* 30: e189–e196.

Rochon, C., Tauveron, I., Dejax, C., et al. (2003) Response of glucose disposal to hyperinsulinaemia in human hypothyroidism and hyperthyroidism. *Clinical Science* 104(1): 7–15.

Rodin, G., Olmsted, M.P., Rydall, A.C., et al. (2002) Eating behaviour in obese patients with and without Type 2 diabetes mellitus. *International Journal of Obesity-Related Metabolic Disorders* 26: 848–853.

Rothwell, P.M., Howard, S.C., Dolan, E., et al. (2010) Prognostic significance of visit-to-visit variability, maximum systolic blood pressure, and episodic hypertension. *Lancet* 375: 895–905.

Rubino, F., Kaplan, L.M., Schauer, P.R., et al. (2010) Diabetes Surgery Summit Delegates. The Diabetes Surgery Summit consensus conference: recommendations for the evaluation and use of gastrointestinal surgery to treat Type 2 diabetes mellitus. *Annuls of Surgery* 251: 399–405.

Rubino, F., Forgione, A., Cummings, D.E., et al. (2006a) The mechanism of diabetes control after gastrointestinal bypass surgery reveals a role of the proximal small intestine in the pathophysiology of Type 2 diabetes. *Annuls of Surgery* 244: 741–749.

Rubino, F. (2006b) Bariatric surgery: effects on glucose homeostasis. *Current Opinion in Clinical Nutrition and Metabolic Care* 9: 497–507.

Russell, R.C. (2012) *Diabetic Ketoacidosis*. Seattle, Washington: VSD Publications.

Rush, M.R., Whitebird, R.R., Rush, M.R., et al. (2008) Depression in patients with diabetes: Does it impact clinical goals? *Journal of the American Board of Family Medicine* 21(5): 392–397.

Rutter, M. (2013) Annual Research Review: Resilience: clinical implications. *Journal of Child Psychology and Psychiatry* 54: 474–487.

Rutter, M. (2012) Resilience as a dynamic concept. *Developmental Psychopathology* 24: 335–344.

Rydall, A.C., Rodin, G.M., Olmsted, M.P., et al. (1997) Disordered eating behavior and microvascular complications in young women with insulin-dependent diabetes mellitus. *New England Journal of Medicine* 336: 1849–1854.

Rydén, L., Grant, P.J., Anker, S.D., et al. (2013) The Task Force on diabetes, prediabetes and cardiovascular diseases of the European Society of Cardiology (ESC) and developed in collaboration with the European Association for the Study of Diabetes (EASD). ESC Guidelines on diabetes, pre-diabetes and cardiovascular diseases, developed in collaboration with the EASD. *European Heart Journal* 34: 3035–3087.

Ryff, C.D., Dienberg-Love, G., et al. (2006) Psychological well-being and ill-being: do they have distinct or mirrored biological correlates? *Psychotherapy and Psychosomatics* 75: 85–95.

Sabel, A.L., Rosen, E., Mehler, P. (2014) Severe anorexia nervosa in males: clinical presentations and medical treatment. *Eating Disorders* 22: 209–220.

Sabel, A.L., Gaudiani, J.L., Statland, B. (2013) Hematological abnormalities in severe anorexia nervosa. *Annals of Hematology* 92: 605–613.

Safren, S.A., Gonzalez, J.S., Wexler, D., et al. (2014) A randomised controlled trial of cognitive behavioural therapy (CBT-AD) in patients with uncontrolled Type 2 diabetes. *Diabetes Care* 37(3): 625–633.

Sakar, U., Fisher, L., Schilliner, D. (2006) Is self-efficacy associated with diabetes self-management across race/ethnicity and health literacy? *Diabetes Care* 29(4): 823–829.

Sakyi, K., Survan, P.J., Fombonne, E., et al. (2015) Childhood friendships and psychological difficulties in young adulthood: an 18-year follow-up study. *European Child and Adolescent Psychology* 24(7): 815–826.

Sanchez-Zaldıvar, S., Arias-Horcajadas, F., Gorgojo-Martınez, J.J., et al. (2009) Evolution of psychopathological alterations in patients with morbid obesity after bariatric surgery. *Medicina Clininca* 33(6): 206–212.

Sanne, J.K., Murray-Cramm, J., Nieboer, A.P. (2019) The importance of patient-centred care and co-creation of care for satisfaction with care and physical and social well-being of patients with multi-morbidity in the primary care setting. *BMC Health Service Research* 19, article 13.

Sarwer, D.B., Dilks, R.J., Ritter, S. (2012) *Bariatric Surgery for Weight Loss: Encyclopedia of Body Image and Human Appearance*, vol. 1. San Diego, California: Academic Press.

Sarwar, N., Gao, P., Seshasai, S.R., et al. (2010) Diabetes mellitus, fasting blood glucose concentration, and risk of vascular disease: a collaborative meta-analysis of 102 prospective studies. *Lancet* 375: 2215–2222.

Saydah, S.H., Brancati, F.L., Golden, S.H., et al. (2003) Depressive symptoms and the risk of Type 2 diabetes mellitus in a US sample. *Diabetes Metabolic Research Revised* 19(3): 202–208.

Schauer, D.P., Arterburn, D.E., Livingston, E.H., et al. (2015) Impact of bariatric surgery on life expectancy in severely obese patients with diabetes: a decision analysis. *Annals of Surgery* https://www.ncbi.nlm.nih.gov/pmc/articles/PMC4388039/

Schauer, P.R., Burguera, B., Ikramuddin, S., et al. (2003) Effect of laparoscopic Roux-en Y gastric bypass on Type 2 diabetes mellitus. *Annuls of Surgery* 238: 467–484; discussion 84–85.

Schernthaner, G., Morton, J.M. (2008) Bariatric surgery in patients with morbid obesity and Type 2 diabetes. *Diabetes Care* 31(2): S297–S302.

Schernthaner, G., Grimaldi, A., Di Mario, U. (2004) GUIDE study: double-blind comparison of once-daily gliclazide MR and glimepiride in Type 2 diabetic patients. *European Journal of Clinical Investigation* 34: 535–542.

Schneider, L.K. (2019) Rising suspicion of Addison's disease in patients with Type 1 diabetes. https://www.endocrineweb.com/professional/other-endocrine-disorders/rising-suspicion-addisons-disease-patients-type-1-diabetes

Schofield, C.J., Yu, N., Jain, A.S. (2009) Decreasing amputation rates in patients with diabetes—A population-based study. *Diabetes Medicine*26: 773–777.

Schofield, J.D., Liu, Y., Rao-Balakrishna, P., et al. (2016) Diabetes dyslipidemia. *Diabetes Therapy* 7(2):203–219.

Schwartz, S.A., Weissberg-Benchell, J., Perlmuter, L.C. (2000) Personal control and disordered eating in female adolescents with Type 1 diabetes. *Diabetes Care* 25: 1987–1991.

Schweiger, C., Weiss, R., Keidar, A. (2010) Effect of different bariatric operations on food tolerance and quality of eating. *Obesity Surgery* 20: 1393–1399.

Schwimmer, J.B., Burwinkle, T.M., Varni, V.W. (2003) Health-related quality of life of severely obese children and adolescents. *Journal of the American Medical Association* 289(14): 1813–1819.

Scopinaro, N., Marinari, G., Camerini, G., et al. (2005) 2004 ABS Consensus Conference: Biliopancreatic diversion for obesity: state of the art. *Surgery and Obesity* 1: 317–328.

Segerstrom, S.C., Miller, G.E. (2004) Psychological stress and the human immune system: a meta-analytic study of 30 years of inquiry. *Psychology Bulletin*130: 601–630.

Seligman, M.E. (1975) *Helplessness*. San Francisco: Freeman.

Settineri, S., Frisone, F., Merlo, E.M., et al. (2019) Compliance, adherence, empowerment, and self-management: five words to manifest a relational maladjustment in diabetes self-management. *Journal Multidisciplinary Healthcare* 12: 299–314.

Shaban, C. (2013) Diabulimia: mental health condition or media hyperbole? *Practical Diabetes.* 30(3): 104–105a.

Shah, M. (2020) Charcot arthropathy. https://emedicine.medscape.com/article/1234293- overview

Shan Xing, S., DiPaul, B.A., Le, H.Y., et al. (2011) Failure to fill electronically-prescribed antidepressant medications: a retrospective study. *Primary Care Companion* https://www.ncbi.nlm.nih.gov/pmc/articles/PMC3121212/

Shaw, K.M., Cummings, M.H. (2005) *Diabetes: Chronic Complications*. Second edition, Chichester: John Wiley and Sons Limited.

Sheldon, K.M., Williams, G., Joiner, T. (2000) *Self Determination Theory in the Clinic: Motivating Physical and Mental Health*. New Haven: Yale University Press.

Shibata, S., Saeki, H., Tada, Y. (2009) Serum high molecular weight adiponectin levels are decreased in psoriasis patients. *Journal of Dermatological Science* 55: 62–63.

Shikiar, R., Heffernan, M., Langley, R.G., et al. (2007) Adalimumab treatment is associated with improvement in health-related quality of life in psoriasis: patient-reported outcomes from a phase II randomized controlled trial. *Journal of Dermatology and Treatment* 18: 25–31.

Sikorski, C., Luppa, M., Kaiser, M., et al. (2011) The stigma of obesity in the general public and its implications for public health – a systematic review. *BMC Public Health* https://link.springer.com/article/10.1186/1471-2458-11-661

Simsek, D.G., Aycan, S., Ozen, Z., et al. (2013) Diabetes care, glycemic control, complications, and concomitant autoimmune diseases in children with Type 1 diabetes in Turkey: a multicenter study. *Journal of Clinical Research in Pediatric Endocrinology* 22(5): 20–26.

Sindrup, S.H., Ejlertsen, B., Gjessing, H., et al. (1988) Peripheral nerve function during hyperglycaemic clamping in healthy subjects. *Acta Neurolgica Scandinavia* 78:141–145.

Singer, M.A. (2001) Of mice and men and elephants: metabolic rate sets glomerular filtration rate. *American Journal of Kidney Diseases* 37(1): 164–178.

Singh, H., Gonder-Frederick, L., Schmidt, K., et al. (2014) Assessing hyperglycemia avoidance in people with Type 1 diabetes. *Diabetes Management* 4(3): 263–271.

Sirey, J.A., Bruce, M.L., Aplexopoulos, G.S., et al. (2001a) Stigma as a barrier to recovery: perceived stigma and patient-related severity of illness as predictors of anti-depressant drug adherence. *Psychiatric Services* 52(12): 1615–1620.

Sirey, J., Bruce, M.L., Raue, P., et al. (2001b) Psychological barriers in young and older outpatients with depression as predictors of treatment discontinuation. *American Journal of Psychiatry* 158: 479–481.

Sjöström, C.D., Lissner, L., Wedel, H., et al. (1999) Reduction in incidence of diabetes, hypertension and lipid disturbances after intentional weight loss induced by bariatric surgery: the SOS intervention study. *Obesity Research* 7(5): 477–484.

Skaff, M.M., Mullan, J.T., Almeida, D.M., et al. (2009) Daily negative mood affects fasting glucose in Type 2 diabetes. *Health Psychology* 28: 265–272.

Skinner, T.C., Carey, M.E., Cradock, S., et al. (2010) Depressive symptoms in the first year from diagnosis of Type 2 diabetes: results from the DESMOND trial. *Diabetes Medicine* 27: 965–967.

Skroubis, G., Sakellaropoulos, G., Pouggouras, K., et al. (2002) Comparison of nutritional deficiencies after Roux-en-Y gastric bypass and after biliopancreatic diversion with Roux-en-Y gastric bypass. *Obesity Surgery* 12: 551–558.

Smith, R.W., Korenblum, C., Thacker, K. (2013) Severely elevated transaminases in an adolescent male with anorexia nervosa. *International Journal of Eating Disorders* 46: 751–754.

Smyth, J.M., Arigo, D. (2009) Recent evidence supports emotion regulation interventions for improving health in at-risk and clinical populations. *Current Opinion in Psychiatry* 22: 205–210.

Sniehotta, F.F., Scholz, U., Schwarzer, R. (2005) Bridging the intention-behaviours gap: planning, self-efficacy, and action control in the adoption and maintenance of physical exercise. *Psychology and Health* 20(2): 14–60.

Snoek, F., Pouwer, F., Welch, G.W., et al. (2000) Diabetes-related emotional distress in Dutch and US diabetic patients: cross-cultural validity of the Problem Areas in Diabetes Scale. *Diabetes Care* 23(9):1305–1309.

Snow, V., Lascher, S., Mottur-Pilson, C. (2000) Pharmacologic treatment of acute major depression and dysthymia. *Annals of Internal Medicine* 132(9): 738–742.

Sola, E., Morillas, C., Garzon, S., et al. (2002) Association between diabetic ketoacidosis and thyrotoxicosis. *Acta Diabetologica* 39(4): 235–237.

Sollid, L.M., Qiao, S-W., Anderson, R.P., et al. (2012) Nomenclature and listing of celiac disease relevant gluten T-cell epitopes restricted by HLA-DQ molecules. *Immunogenetics* 64(6): 455–460.

Sommerfield, A.J., Deary, I.J., Frier, B.M. (2004) Acute hyperglycaemia alters mood state and impairs cognitive performance in people with Type 2 diabetes. *Diabetes Care* 27: 2335–2340.

Sowunmi, A. (1993) Psychosis after cerebral malaria in children. *Journal of the National Medical Association* 85: 695–696.

Spadaccino, A.C., Basso, D., Chiarelli, S., et al. (2008) Celiac disease in North Italian patients with autoimmune thyroid diseases. *Autoimmunity* 41(1): 116–121.

Speight, J., Browne, J.L., Holmes-Truscott, E., et al. (2011) Diabetes MILES (Management and Impact of Long-term Empowerment and Success) Australia: methods and sample characteristics of a national survey of the psychological aspects of living with Type 1 or Type 2 diabetes in Australian adults. Canberra: Diabetes Australia.

Spelman, L.M., Walsh, P.I., Sharifi, N., et al. (2007) Impaired glucose tolerance in first-episode drug-naïve patients with schizophrenia. *Diabetic Medicine* 24: 481–485.

Sponzilli, I., Chiari, G., Iovane, B., et al. (2010) Celiac disease in children with Type 1 diabetes: impact of gluten-free diet on diabetes management. *Acta Biomedica* 81(3): 165–170.

Sporns, O. (2011) *Networks of the Brain*. Cambridge, Massachusetts: MIT Press.

Stagi, S., Giani, T., Simonini, G., et al. (2005) Thyroid function, autoimmune thyroiditis and coeliac disease in juvenile idiopathic arthritis. *Rheumatology* 44 (4): 517–520.

Stanton-Fey, S.H., Hamilton, K., Chadwick, P.M., et al. (2021) The DAFNE*plus* programme for sustained Type 1 diabetes self-management: intervention development using the Behaviour Change Wheel. *Diabetic Medicine* e14548. 10.1111/dme.14548. (In press).

Starkey, K. & Wade, T. (2010) Disordered eating in girls with Type 1 diabetes: examining directions for prevention. *Clinical Psychologist* 14(1): 2–9.

Steenkamp, D., Patel, V., Minkin, R. (2011) A case of pneumomediastinum: a rare complication of diabetes. *Clinical Diabetes* 29(2): 76–77.

Steinhardt, M.A., Mamerow, M.M., Brown, S.A., et al. (2009) A resilience intervention in African American adults with Type 2 diabetes: a pilot study of efficacy. *Diabetes Educator* 35: 274–284.

Sterry, W., Strober, B.E., Menter, A. (2007) Obesity in psoriasis: the metabolic, clinical and therapeutic implications. Report of an interdisciplinary conference and review. *British Journal of Dermatology* 157: 649–655.

Sterry, W., Strober, B.E., Menter, A. (2007) Obesity in psoriasis: the metabolic, clinical and therapeutic implications. Report of an interdisciplinary conference and review. *British Journal of Dermatology* 157: 649–655.

Stratton, I.M., Adler, A.I., Neil, H.A., et al. (2000) Association of glycaemia with macrovascular and microvascular complications of Type 2 diabetes (UKPDS 35): prospective observational study. *British Medical Journal* 21: 405–412.

Strumia, R. (2005) Dermatologic signs in patients with eating disorders. *American Journal of Clinical Dermatology* 6: 1–10.

Stuckey, H.L., Mullan-Jensen, C.B., Reach, G., et al. (2014) Personal accounts of the negative and adaptive psychosocial experiences of people with diabetes in the second Diabetes Attitudes, Wishes and Needs (DAWN2) study. *Diabetes Care* 37: 2466–2474.

Subramanian, A., Adderley, N.J., Tracy, A., et al. (2019) Risk of incident obstructive sleep apnoea among patients with Type 2 Diabetes. *Diabetes Care* 42(5): 954–963.

Sullivan, M.D., Katon, W.J., Lovato, L.C., et al. (2013) Association of depression with accelerated cognitive decline among patients with Type 2 diabetes in the ACCORD-MIND trial. *Journal of the American Medical Association of Psychiatry* 70: 1041–1047.

Sun, J.K., Keenan, H.A., Cavallarano, J.D., et al, (2011) Protection from retinopathy and other complications in patients with Type 1 diabetes of extreme duration. *Diabetes Care* 34: 968–974.

Svenson, M., Engström, I., Aman, J., et al. (2003) Higher drive for thinness in adolescent males with insulin-dependent diabetes mellitus compared with healthy controls. *Acta Paediatrica* 12: 122–128.

Swanson, V., Maltinsky, W. (2019) Motivational and behavioural change approaches for improving diabetes management. *Practical Diabetes* https://www.practicaldiabetes.com/article/motivational-and-behaviour-change-approaches-for-improving-diabetes-management/

Taguchi, S., Oinuma, T., Yamada, T. (2000) A comparative study of cultured smooth muscle cell proliferation and injury, utilizing glycated low-density lipoproteins with slight oxidation, auto-oxidation, or extensive oxidation. *Journal of Atherosclerosis and Thrombosis* 7: 132–137.

Takahashi, H., Tsuji, H., Takahashi, I., et al. (2008) Plasma adiponectin and leptin levels in Japanese patients with psoriasis. *British Journal of Dermatology* 159: 1207–1208.

Talbot, F., Nouwen, A. (2000) A review of the relationship between depression and diabetes in adults: is there a link? *Diabetes Care* 23: 1556–1562.

Tam, L.S., Tomlinson, B., Chu, T.T., et al. (2008) Cardiovascular risk profile of patients with psoriatic arthritis compared to controls–the role of inflammation. *Rheumatology* 47: 718–723.

Tamer, E., Gur, G., Polat, M., et al. (2009) Flare-up of pustular psoriasis with Fluoxetine: possibility of a serotoninergic influence? *Journal of Dermatology Treatment* 20: 137–140.

Temneanu, O.R., Trandafir, L.M., Purcarea, M.R. (2016) Type 2 diabetes mellitus in children and adolescents: a relatively new clinical problem within paediatric practice.

Tan Pei Lin, L., Kwek, S.K. (2010) Onset of psoriasis during therapy with Fluoxetine. *General Hospital Psychiatry* 32: 446: e9–e10.

Titchner, J. (2020) A patient-centred clinical approach to diabetes care assists long-term reduction in HbA1c. *Journal of Primary Health Care* 6(3): 195–202.

The Mental Health Foundation (2020) Mental health statistics: UK and worldwide. https://www.mentalhealth.org.uk/statistics/mental-health-statistics-uk-and-worldwide#:~:text=Major%20depression%20is%20thought%20to,suicide%20and%20ischemic%20heart%20disease

Thoolen, B.J., de Ridder, D., Bensing, J., et al. (2009) Beyond good intentions: the role of proactive coping in achieving sustained behavioural change in the context of diabetes management. *Psychology and Health* 24: 237–254.

Tiberti, C., Panimolle, P., Bonamico, M., et al. (2012) IgA antitransglutaminase autoantibodies at Type 1 diabetes onset are less frequent in adult patients and are associated with a general celiac-specific lower immune response in comparison with non-diabetic celiac patients at diagnosis. *Diabetes Care* 35(10): 2083–2085.

Timonen, M., Laakso, M., Jokelainen, J., et al. (2005) Insulin resistance and depression: cross-sectional study. *British Medical Journal* 330:17–18, 2005.

Tobin, A.M., Veale, D.J., Fitzgerald, O., et al. (2010) Cardiovascular disease and risk factors in patients with psoriasis and psoriatic arthritis. *Journal of Rheumatology* 37: 1386–1394.

Triolo, T.M., Armstrong, T.K., McFann, K., et al. (2011) Additional autoimmune disease found in 33% of patients at Type 1 diabetes onset. *Diabetes Care* 34 (5): 1211–1213.

Tsai, A.G., Wadden, T.A. (2005) Systematic review: an evaluation of major commercial weight loss programs in the United States. *Annuls of Intern Medicine* 142: 56–66.

Tseng, C.L., Soroka, O., Maney, M. (2014) Assessing potential glycemic over-treatment in persons at hypoglycemic risk. *Journal of the American Medical Association Internal Medicine* 174: 259–268.

Tsukayama, E., Toomey, S.L., Faith, M.S., et al. (2010) Self-control as a protective factor against overweight status in the transition from childhood to adolescence. *Archive of Pediatric and Adolescent Medicine* 164: 631–635.

UCLA (2020) Acute Adrenal Crisis (Addisonian crisis). https://www.uclahealth.org/endocrine-center/acute-adrenal-crisis

UKPDS Group (1998a) Intensive blood glucose control with sulfonylureas or insulin compared with conventional treatment and risk of complications in patients with Type 2 diabetes (UKPDS 33). *Lancet* 352: 837–853.

UKPDS Group (1998b) Effect of intensive blood glucose control with Metformin on complications in overweight patients with Type 2 diabetes (UKPDS 34). *Lancet* 352: 854–865.

UKPDS Group (1998c) Tight blood pressure control and risk of macrovascular and microvascular complications in Type 2 diabetes: UKPDS 38. Prospective Diabetes Study Group.

Ulger, Z., Gürses, D., Ozyurek, A.R. (2006) Follow-up of cardiac abnormalities in female adolescents with anorexia nervosa after refeeding. *Acta Cardiology* 61: 43–49.

Utiger, R.D. (1995) Altered thyroid function in nonthyroidal illness and surgery. To treat or not to treat? *New England Journal of Medicine* 7: 1562–1563.

Uysal, A.R., Erdogan, M.F., Sahin, G., et al. (1998) Clinical and metabolic effects of fasting in 41 Type 2 diabetic patients during Ramadan (Letter). *Diabetes Care* 21: 2033–2034.

Vahdat, S., Hamzehgardeshi, L., Hessam, S., et al. (2014) Patient involvement in health care decision making: a review. *Iranian Red Crescent Medical Journal* https://www.ncbi.nlm.nih.gov/pmc/articles/PMC3964421/

Valerio, G., Spadaro, R., Iafusco, D., et al. (2008) The influence of gluten free diet on quantitative ultrasound of proximal phalanxes in children and adolescents with Type 1 diabetes mellitus and celiac disease. *Bone* 43(2): 322–326.

Van Bastelaar, K.M.P., Pouwer, F., Cuijpers, P., et al. (2008) Web-based cognitive behavioural therapy (W-CBT) for diabetes patients with co-morbid depression: design of a randomised-controlled trial. *British Medical Council of Psychiatry* https://link.springer.com/article/10.1186/1471-244X-8-9

Van de Laar, F.A., Lucassen, P.L., Akkermans, R.P., et al. (2005) Alpha-glucosidase inhibitors for Type 2 diabetes mellitus. *Cochrane Database Systematic Review* CD003639.

Vander Wal, J.S., Mitchell, E.R. (2011) Psychological complications of pediatric obesity. *Clinics of North America* 58(6): 1393–1401.

Van Hout, G.C.M., Boekestein, P., Fortuin, F.A.M., et al. (2006) Psychosocial functioning following bariatric surgery. *Obesity Surgery* 16(6): 787–794.

Van Hout, G.C.M. (2005) Psychosocial effects of bariatric surgery. *Acta Chirurgica Belgica* 105(1): 40–43. *Gastroenterology and Nutrition* 56(6): 663–670.

Van Servellen, G., Heise, B.A., Ellis, R. (2011) Factors associated with anti-depressant medication adherence-enhancement programmes: a systematic literature review. *Mental Health in Family Medicine* 8(4): 255–271.

Vaxilliare, M., Froguel, P. (2010) The genetics of Type 2 diabetes from candidate gene biology to genome-wide studies. In: Holt, R.I.G., et al. (Eds.) *Textbook of Diabetes.* Oxford: Wiley-Blackwell.

Verhoeven, E.W., Kraaimaat, F.W., de Jong, E.M., et al. (2009a) Effect of daily stressors on psoriasis: a prospective study. *Journal of Investigation into Dermatology* 129: 2075–2077.

Verhoeven, E.W., Kraaimaat, F.W., de Jong, E.M., et al. (2009b) Individual differences in the effect of daily stressors on psoriasis: a prospective study. *British Journal of Dermatology* 161: 295–299.

Vernon MC, Mavropoulos J, Transue M, et al. (2003) Clinical experience of a carbohydrate-restricted diet: effect on diabetes mellitus. *Metabolic Syndrome and Related Disorders* 1: 233–238.

Vileikyte, L., Leventhal, H., Gonzalez, J., et al. (2005) Diabetic peripheral neuropathy and depressive symptoms. *Diabetes Care* 28: 2378–2383.

Viljamada, M., Kaukinen, K., Huhtala, H., et al. (2005) Coeliac disease, autoimmune diseases and gluten exposure. *Scandinavian Journal of Gastroenterology* 40(4): 437–443.

Viljoen, A. (2011) Investigating mixed hyperlipidaemia. *British Medical Journal* 343: d5146.

Vohs, K.D., Faber, R.J. (2007) Spent resources: self-regulatory resource availability affects impulse buying. *Journal of Consumer Research* 33: 537–547.

Wagner, J., Tsimikis, J., Abbott, G., et al. (2007) Racial and ethnic differences in diabetic patient-reported depression symptoms, diagnosis, and treatment. *Diabetes Research and Clinical Practice* 75(1): 119–122.

Walker, J.D., Young, R.J., Little, J., et al. (2002) Mortality in concurrent Type 1 diabetes and anorexia nervosa. *Diabetes Care* 25(9): 1571–1575.

Walker, R.J., Smalls, B.L., Hernandez-Tejada, M.A., et al. (2012) Effect of diabetes fatalism on medication adherence and self-care behaviors in adults with diabetes. *General Hospital Psychiatry* 34: 598–603.

Wang, Y., Chen, J., Zhao, Y., et al. (2008) Psoriasis is associated with increased levels of serum leptin. *British Journal of Dermatology* 158: 1134–1135.

Walter, R.E., Beiser, A., Givelber, R.J., et al. (2003) Association between glycemic state and lung function: the Framingham Heart Study. *American Journal of Respiration and Critical Care Medicine* 167: 911–916.

Wax, R. (2013) *Sane New World: Taming The Mind.* Croydon: Hodder & Stoughton.

Webb, T.L., Sheeran, P. (2003) Can implementation intentions help to overcome ego-depletion? *Journal of Experimental and Social Psychology* 39: 279–286.

Weiden, P., Olfson, M., Essock, S. (1997) Medication noncompliance in schizophrenia: effects on mental health service policy. In: *Treatment Compliance and the Therapeutic Alliance: Chronic Mental Illness,* volume 5. Blackwell, B. (Ed.), Singapore: Harwood Academic.

Weiss, S.C., Kimball, A.B., Liewehr, D.J., et al. (2002) Quantifying the harmful effect of psoriasis on health-related quality of life. *Journal of American Academic Dermatology* 47: 512–518.

Weissman, M.M., Bland, R.C., Canino, G.J., et al. (1996) Cross-national epidemiology of major depression and bipolar disorder. *Journal of the American Medical Association* 276: 293–299.

West, R. and Michie, S. (2020) A brief introduction to the COM-B Model of behaviour and the PRIME Theory of motivation. *Qeios* https://www.qeios.com/read/WW04E6.2

West, R. (2006) *Theory of Addiction.* Oxford: Blackwell Publishing.

Westman, E.C., Yancy, W.S., Mavropoulos, J.C., et al. (2008) The effect of a low-carbohydrate, ketogenic diet versus a low glycaemic index diet on glycaemic control in Type 2 diabetes mellits. *Nutrition and Metabolism* 5: 36.

Whitlock, G., Lewington, S., Sherliker, P., et al. (2009) Body-mass index and cause-specific mortality in 900,000 adults: collaborative analyses of 57 prospective studies. *Lancet* 373 (9669): 1083–1096.

Willey, K.A., Singh, M.A. (2003) Battling insulin resistance in elderly obese people with Type 2 diabetes: bring on the heavy weights. *Diabetes Care* 26:1580–1588.

Williams, J.S., Walker, R.J., Smalls, B.L., et al. (2016) Patient-centred care, glycaemic control, diabetes self-care, and quality of life in adults with Type 2 diabetes. *Diabetes Technology and Therapeutics* 18(10): 644–649.

Williams, M.W., Clouse, R.E., Lustman, P.J. (2006) Understanding depression as a medical risk factor to prevent diabetes and its complications. *Clinical Diabetes* 24(2): 79–89.

Willis T. (1675) *Pharmaceutice rationalis sive diabtriba de medicamentorum operantionibus in humano corpore.* Oxford.

Wilson, V.L. (2019) *How To Live Well with Diabetes: A Comprehensive Guide to Taking Control of Your Life with Diabetes.* London: Robinson; Little Brown Book Group.

Wilson, V.L. (2014) *Insulin: Uses and Abuses.* New York: Teneo Press.

Wilson, V.L. (2012) Reflections on reducing insulin to lose weight. *Nursing Times* 108(43): 21-25.

Wilson, V.L. (2009) Behavioural change in Type 1 diabetes self-management: why and how? *Health Education Journal* 68(4): 320–327.

Wilson, V.L. (2005) Insulin Pump Therapy. In: *Structured Patient Education in Diabetes: Report from the Patient Education Working Group.* London: Department of Health/Diabetes UK.

Wilson, V.L. (2004a) Gastroparesis: a patient's experience. *Journal of Diabetes Nursing* 8(2): 73–75.

Wilson, V.L. (2004b) The NSF for Diabetes: addressing psychosocial issues. *Journal of Diabetes Nursing* 8(10): 372–376.

Wilson, V.L. (2003) Survey of information and support needs of people with Type 1 diabetes. *Journal of Diabetes Nursing* 7(7): 272–277.

Wisting, L., Bang, L., Skrivarhaug, T., et al. (2015) Adolescents with T1D – The impact of gender, age, and health-related functioning on eating disorder psychopathology. *PLoS ONE* 10(11): e0141386.

Wooley, S.C., Garner, D.M. (1991) Obesity treatment: the high cost of false hope. *Journal of the American Dietetic Association* 91(10): 1248–1251.

World Health Organization (2021) Global InfoBase *International Comparisons* https://apps.who.int/infobase/Comparisons.aspx?l=&NodeVal=WGIE_BMI_5_cd.0704&.

Worthy, D.A., Byrne, K.A., Fields, S. (2014) Effects of emotion on prospection during decision-making. *Frontiers of Psychology* 5: 591. doi: 10.3389/fpsyg.2014.00591

Yang, G.R., Yang, J.K., Zhang, L., et al. (2010) Association between subclinical hypothyroidism and proliferative diabetic retinopathy in Type 2 diabetic patients: a case-control study. *Tokyo Journal of Experimental Medicine* 222(4): 303–310.

Yanling, W., Yanping, D., Yoshimasa, T., et al. (2016) Risk factors contributing to Type 2 diabetes and recent advances in treatment and prevention. *International Journal of Medical Sciences* 11(11): 1185–1200.

Yashuhara, D., Deguchi, D., Tsutsui, J. (2003) Reactive hypoglycemia induced by rapid change in eating behavior in anorexia nervosa. *International Journal of Eating Disorders* 34: 273–277.

Yi-Frazier, J.P., Smith, R.E., Vitaliano, P.P., et al. (2010) A person-focused analysis of resilience resources and coping in diabetes patients. *Stress and Health* 26: 51–60.

Young, V., Eiser, C., Johnson, B., et al. (2013) Eating problems in adolescents with Type 1 diabetes: a systematic review with meta-analysis. *Diabetes Medicine* 30: 189–198.

Young-Hyman, D.L., Davis, C.L. (2010) *Disordered Eating in Individuals with Diabetes: Importance of Context, Evaluation and Classification.* American Diabetes Association http://creativecommons.org/licenses/by-nc-nd/3.0/

Yung-Tsung, H., Wen-Chien, C., Wei-Chih, L., et al. (2015) Type 1 diabetes and increased risk of subsequent asthma: a nationwide population-based cohort study. *Medicine* 94(36): pe1466.

Zeller, M.H., Reiter-Purtill, J., Ratcliff, M.B., et al. (2011) Two-year trends in psychosocial functioning after adolescent Roux-en-Y gastric bypass. *Surgery for Obesity and Related Diseases* 7(6): 727–732.

Zeller, M.H., Roehrig, H.R., Modi, A.C., et al. (2006) Health-related quality of life and depressive symptoms in adolescents with extreme obesity presenting for bariatric surgery. *Pediatrics* 117, (4): 1155–1161.

Index

For Product Safety Concerns and Information please contact our EU
representative GPSR@taylorandfrancis.com Taylor & Francis Verlag GmbH,
Kaufingerstraße 24, 80331 München, Germany

Printed and bound by CPI Group (UK) Ltd, Croydon, CR0 4YY
08/06/2025
01897006-0001